Nursing Case Management

An Evolving Practice

Notice

Medicine is an ever-changing science. As new research and clinical experience broaden our knowledge, changes in treatment and drug therapy are required. The authors and the publisher of this work have checked with sources believed to be reliable in their efforts to provide information that is complete and generally in accord with the standards accepted at the time of publication. However, in view of the possibility of human error or changes in medical sciences, neither the authors nor the publisher nor any other party who has been involved in the preparation or publication of this work warrants that the information contained herein is in every respect accurate or complete, and they are not responsible for any errors or omissions or for the results obtained from use of such information. Readers are encouraged to confirm the information contained herein with other sources. For example and in particular, readers are advised to check the product information sheet included in the package of each drug they plan to administer to be certain that the information contained in this book is accurate and that changes have not been made in the recommended dose or in the contraindications for administration. This recommendation is of particular importance in connection with new or infrequently used drugs.

Nursing Case Management

An Evolving Practice

PHYLLIS K. MORE, PhD, RNC

PROFESSOR OF NURSING

Bloomfield College
Division of Nursing
Bloomfield, New Jersey

SANDY MANDELL, MA, CRRN, CIRS, CCM

Director, Case Management Services
Dimensions in Managed Care
Montville, New Jersey

New York   St. Louis   San Francisco   Auckland   Bogotá   Caracas

Lisbon   London   Madrid   Mexico City   Milan   Montreal

New Delhi   San Juan   Singapore   Sydney   Tokyo   Toronto

McGraw-Hill
Health
Professions
Division

McGraw-Hill

A Division of The **McGraw·Hill** *Companies*

Nursing Case Management: An Evolving Practice

Copyright © 1997 by The McGraw-Hill Companies, Inc. All rights reserved. Printed in the United States of America. Except as permitted under the United States Copyright Act of 1976, no part of this publication may be reproduced or distributed in any form or by any means, or stored in a data base or retrieval system, without the prior written permission of the publisher.

234567890   DOCDOC   987

ISBN 0-07-105481-2

This book was set in Perpetua by V&M Graphics, Inc.
The editors were Gail Gavert and Peter McCurdy;
the production supervisor was Rick Ruzycka;
the cover designer was Patrice Sheridan.
Irving Tullar prepared the index.
R.R. Donnelley & Sons was printer and binder.

This book is printed on acid-free paper.

LIBRARY OF CONGRESS CATALOGING-IN-PUBLICATION DATA

More, Phyllis K.
    Case management : an evolving practice / Phyllis K. More, Sandy
Mandell.
        p.   cm.
    Includes bibliographical references and index.
    ISBN 0-07-105481-2
    1. Hospitals—United States—Case management services.   2. Primary
nursing—United States.   3. Managed care plans (Medical care)—
United States.   I. Mandell, Sandy.   II. Title.
RA975.5.C36M67   1996
362.1′73′068—dc20   96-13465

Contents

APPENDICES

Preface

"*The fundamental assumptions on which nursing knowledge and nursing practice rest are being rewritten by the very terms of man's existence. People are at the center of nursing's purpose. The descriptive, explanatory, and predictive principles that direct professional nursing practice are rooted in a fundamental concept of the wholeness of life.*"[1]

MARTHA E. ROGERS (1970)

Nursing case management is often viewed as a relatively new idea, a concept that emerged out of the need to resolve the increasing cost of health care and that continues to evolve into an holistic approach to patient care. Case management decreases fragmentation, increases quality and has become a significant link connecting the client and the health care delivery system.

In reality, nurses have been providing a variety of case management services since the turn of the century. Early public health nurses established a connection between members of the community and health care services. These nurses provided direct care, educated clients, referred them to other resources and assumed responsibility for the overall management of the client. In this way,

---

[1]Rogers, M. (1970). *An introduction to the theoretical basis of nursing.* Philadelphia: FA Davis. 34.

nursing's tradition as coordinators of care and client advocates became established. As the nursing profession evolved to demand higher levels of education and establish a base for independent practice, nurses gained increased responsibility, and they acquired greater power and authority. As with all things, change begets change. Case management, seen by many as a new role, was in fact a redefinition and restructuring of an already existing practice strategy.

Rapid shifts in the health care delivery system have generated increasing interest in mechanisms for delivery of high quality, cost-effective care. A major outcome of this trend has been the emergence of case management as a model for organizing care in a variety of settings. While numerous disciplines have staked a claim as case managers, nursing is without doubt the profession with the most appropriate knowledge base and skill base to prepare competent case managers.

As a model of health care delivery, case management has developed from "the bottom up." The desire for cost savings and retention of "a piece of the health care pie" has inspired nurses to develop skill in case management. For the most part, the knowledge base they require has been developed through personal experience, trial and error, networking, conferences, and a very limited amount of interdisciplinary literature dedicated to this area of practice.

This book has been developed as a traditional text. It is designed to provide the foundational scope and breadth of information for the nurse with minimal exposure to the role of the nurse case manager. Although intended as a resource for the undergraduate and graduate nursing student, the content is equally relevant for the nurse new to the role of case manager.

Since much of case management is concerned with cost containment and cost effectiveness, it is imperative that the reader comprehend the complexities of health care financing. Managed care, which has become increasingly entrenched in health care delivery is discussed in general terms, with emphasis placed on defining the changing role of the case manager working within the limits of a managed care system. Traditional indemnity and workers' compensation insurance are also discussed for comparison and clarity.

Communication is the mainstay of successful case management. Equally important are the various personal and interpersonal skills needed for case managers to function effectively. These skills are explored in depth using a clearly developed classification model. Each skill is examined separately, with specific examples of how it would be used within the case management process to bring about positive outcomes.

Internal and external case management are described in detail. The history, development, and continuing evolution of case management across the continuum of care are compared and contrasted. The various models of case management are discussed and organized in a clear and succinct manner which explains how they evolved. Critical pathways are discussed from their inception through the current trend of required usage in conjunction with continuous quality improvement.

The process of case management is explored using a nursing process approach. Case management is conceptually akin to the nursing process in that both are predicated on a model of problem solving. The specific steps of the case management process are thoroughly covered, with an emphasis on adhering to the standards of practice recently developed by the Case Management Society of America.

Certain populations requiring case management services such as clients diagnosed with HIV/AIDS, mental illness, high-risk pregnancies, severe congenital anomalies or young children or young adults with spinal cord injuries have inherent special needs. The issues are dealt with specific to each diagnosis with recommendations for successful case management.

As nurses and nurse case managers are becoming more autonomous, they are facing a greater array of professional, ethical, and legal issues. These issues are examined in order to sensitize the beginning or experienced practitioner to the many influences affecting practice. Furthermore, understanding of such issues is essential if nurse case managers are to be change agents in this rapidly evolving profession. Many of the legal issues are presented in light of the standards of practice for case managers, which have not yet been tested in any court of law. The reader is provided with guidelines to reduce liability risks.

Lifecare planning is a critical element in maximizing healthcare resources for the client experiencing catastrophic illness or injury. In light of caps on insurance benefits, and/or situations where the client is involved in litigation, the nurse case manager must be equipped with the knowledge to plan for efficient allocation of monies to best ensure ability to provide care for the expected lifespan.

Seven appendices provide supplemental information of use to any case manager. Several examples of reports, the essential documentation tool for the case manager, are included. Differences between documentation for the client with traditional indemnity insurance or workers' compensation insurance are explored, using easy to understand examples. A thorough and complete list of resources, with internet addresses when available, is listed in a format affording ease of identification. Case manager certification exams are discussed, with emphasis on eligibility requirements, exam categories and information pertaining to maintaining certification. A list of professional organizations and suggested journals is reviewed with mailing addresses for additional information. Examples of critical pathways are included to enhance comprehension and appreciation for this newly developed format for multidisciplinary care planning. To assist the reader in integrating the material presented within the contents of the book, a week in the life of a case manager has been developed, using an easy to read format.

We believe that since nursing case management has become an integral component of healthcare delivery, it now must also be incorporated into nursing curricula. *Nursing Case Management: An Evolving Practice* was written to meet the needs of today's students who will be the nurse case managers of the twenty-first century.

We are grateful for the support offered by family and colleagues. We are especially indebted to Gail Gavert, our editor at McGraw-Hill who provided the encouragement and technical assistance to bring this book from concept to reality.

Why Case 1
Management

"It was the best of times, it was the worst of times . . ." wrote Charles Dickens in *A Tale of Two Cities*. Although written more than a century ago, and describing socioeconomic and political conditions of a society quite different from the United States today, the words still ring true when we reflect on current conditions in our health care system.

A SYSTEM IN CRISIS

The U.S. health care system is considered by many to be the premiere system of the world. We have the highest ratio of health care providers per person, the most innovative and sophisticated technology for diagnosis and treatment, and the largest number of treatment facilities. In areas of *secondary prevention* (early diagnosis and treatment of disease), and *tertiary prevention* (reducing consequences of illness and initiating rehabilitation), few countries' outcomes surpass ours. The substantial number of residents of foreign countries who travel to the United States in search of the best and newest treatments attest to the excellence of our system. Our own population has come to expect only the best that medical science can offer. For these reasons, we could assert that, indeed, these are the "best of times" for delivery of complex health care services to an enormous, heterogeneous, and consuming population.

However, this presents only one side of the story. Although we do excel in the quality and quantity of services, the development of a sophisticated and excellent health care system has been very costly. And so, although health care in this country is outstanding in terms of quality, it has also become prohibitively expensive. In the past three decades, the interaction of social forces, legislation, development of new technologies, and changing morbidity patterns have created ever increasing demand for health care services for which costs have skyrocketed. Health care, which consumed only 5.0 percent of the gross domestic product (GDP) in 1965,[1] now accounts for almost 15 percent of the GDP and is expected to account for 18 percent of the GDP by the year 2000.[2] A large segment of our population, estimated at about 40 million, is either uninsured or underinsured and cannot access even the most basic health care services.

Perhaps even more problematic is the very nature of the structure of the U.S. health care system—it is pluralistic, multicentric, and fragmented.[3] *Pluralistic* means that many complementary as well as competing agencies in both the public and private sector have been established to deliver health care. *Multicentric* means that decisions regarding health care are arrived at from many different components of the system, and no single agency is responsible for establishing a national health care policy or agenda. *Fragmentation* is the outcome of the prior two characteristics. Lack of unity in decision making and delivery results in duplication of some services and large gaps in others. These factors might encourage us to believe that the health care system is confronting "the worst of times." We have a complex, highly technological system that has the potential to deliver enormous quantities of quality care to the population. At the same time, we have an underserved component of the population, excessive costs, and serious fragmentation. Leading social commentators assert that the system is in crisis.

It was in this context that private insurance companies introduced the practice of *external case management* in the 1970s. Their goal was to develop a strategy for controlling very expensive claims, usually created by catastrophic accident or illness, and at the same time ensure high-quality care. By the mid 1980s, hospitals began to feel the same financial pinch due to changing structures of reimbursement for their services. And so hospitals sought to develop alternative strategies for delivering care as they were forced to achieve satisfactory patient outcomes in a controlled period of time and with restricted resources. Thus, the role of *internal* (or "within-the-walls") *case manager* began to evolve. Today, case management is a component of virtually all health care delivery systems.

THE ROLE OF THE NURSE CASE MANAGER

Nurse case managers are catalysts and facilitators responsible for coordinating high-quality care in a time-effective, cost-effective manner across the continuum of health care. Case management is a collaborative and multidisciplinary process that closely parallels the framework of the nursing process. The nursing process has been widely accepted as a systematic method for assessing an individual's health status, diagnosing needs, developing a plan of care, implementing the plan, and evaluating the outcomes of the plan.[4]

The process of case management is more global than the nursing process. Case management includes additional components of case selection; multidisciplinary assessment; collective planning; coordinating; negotiating; evaluating; and documenting the outcomes in terms of cost and quality as well as client status. In addition to assisting the client with health care needs, the case management process includes vocational, motivational, and financial strategies.

PROFESSIONAL ORGANIZATIONS' DEFINITIONS OF CASE MANAGEMENT

Many professionals in different disciplines practice some form of case management. Each discipline has developed a definition of *case management* that is specific to that discipline. There are over 100,000 professional case managers, of whom over 15,000 are certified.[5] Nurses, social workers, and vocational counselors represent the largest number of case managers. The following are the definitions used by the Individual Case Management Association (ICMA), the Case Management Society of America (CMSA), and the Association of Rehabilitation Nurses (ARN). The American Nurses Association (ANA) has not yet established a concise definition of case management; however, it advocates eight characteristics of a nurse case manager (discussed below).

ICMA and CMSA

ICMA and CMSA both endorse the following definition: "Case management is a collaborative process which assesses, plans, implements, coordinates, monitors and evaluates options and services to meet an individual's health needs through communication and available resources to promote quality cost-effective outcomes."[6]

ICMA was formed in 1989 to provide leadership and educational support for the growing numbers of case managers. As the first national organization dedicated to promoting and supporting case management, the ICMA was instrumental in developing a national certification program for the case manager (CCM, Certified Case Manager). Members of this organization include nurse case managers as well as social workers and vocational counselors.

CMSA was founded in 1990 to recognize case management on a national level and to share information and promote professional growth. In June, 1996 both organizations merged to consolidate their efforts into one nonprofit organization. As of this writing, the organizations have a combined total of approximately 7300 members.

The agendas of both organizations are tailored for the case managers outside the acute care facility. At this time no national hospital-based case management organization exists. Some regional organizations have sprung up to recognize, promote, and share knowledge among the nurse case managers in acute care. One such organization, established in February 1995, is the Hospital Based Case Manager (HBCM), covering the state of Wisconsin, with approximately 125 members. According to Sue Samrow, one of the founders of HBCM, they have not developed a standard definition of case management because the interpretation is different from institution to institution based upon the needs of the specific facility.[7] The first hospital case management conference was held in the Spring of 1996.

ARN

ARN defines case management as "the process of planning, organizing, coordinating and monitoring the services and resources needed to respond to an individual's health care needs."[8] As the national organization for nurses employed in the field of rehabilitation, ARN was founded in 1974. Most members are "hands-on" rehabilitation nurses, with a growing population of case managers working within the insurance industry. ARN developed the national certification exam for the rehabilitation nurse (CRRN, Certified Rehabilitation Registered Nurse).

ANA

With 200,000 members, the ANA is the national organization for all registered nurses regardless of area of practice or specialty. Although the ANA has not established a specific definition of case management, it has described the following as characteristics for nurses involved in case management. The nurse case manager:

1. Is client focused
2. Is outcome oriented
3. Facilitates and promotes coordination of care and minimizes fragmentation
4. Is cost-effective

5. Collaborates with all members of the health care team
6. Responds to the needs of insurers
7. Represents a merger of clinical and financial interests
8. Plays a role in marketing strategies of hospitals[9]

As the concept of case management has infiltrated almost every aspect of health care, accurately defining the term has become more complex. A clear definition must incorporate the essence of case management across all disciplines and include all models. As case management continues to evolve, and as the different branches of the profession become unified, the definitions are likely to become more precise and comprehensive.

COMPONENTS OF CASE MANAGEMENT

The case manager establishes a partnership with the client with the goal of ensuring optimum cost-effective outcomes. The case manager plays three distinct roles: a case facilitator, an educator of the client system, and an advocate. The case manager ensures coordinated and cost-effective care from various providers. She or he teaches the client about the illness or injury, the health care delivery system, community resources, insurance benefits, and other related issues to enhance client wellness and to ensure that the client can make informed decisions. Because the case manager coordinates services with various providers of care, resources are used efficiently. The case manager acts in the best interest of the client to ensure safety and well being.[10]

Skills of the Nurse Case Manager

The ANA outlines various skills that the case manager must possess. These skills are consistent regardless of the nature of the client problem or of the setting which employs the case manager. These skills include:

- Case finding and screening
- Comprehensive health assessment
- Assessment of support systems
- Analysis and synthesis of health care data to formulate appropriate interdisciplinary problem statements
- Modification of the plan of care through interdisciplinary and collaborative team processes
- Linkage of patients with appropriate resources
- Coordination of service providers
- Education of the client, family, and community support systems concerning the value of self-care of the client
- Monitoring the client's progress toward goal achievement
- Monitoring the service plan to ensure services are appropriate and cost-effective
- Evaluation of client and program outcomes to determine if the client should be discharged or assigned an inactive status[11]

In 1995, the CMSA developed standards of practice specifically for the case manager. These standards serve to educate the public regarding the functions and roles of a case manager, document professional standards that should be adhered to for the purpose of maintaining the highest quality of care, and increase the credibility of the profession. These standards of practice are guidelines for accountability, professionalism, and goals that the case manager aims to achieve.[12] At this time it is unclear whether these standards of practice will be applied regardless of employment setting.

The Purpose of Case Management

Case management is a 24-hour phenomenon. The case manager is the health care provider who ensures the maintenance of the holistic essence of life. The case manager's goals include: continuity of care, cost containment and assurance of appropriate and timely intervention, and smooth transition across the care continuum. These activities reduce fragmentation which may occur, according to M. Clark's *Nursing in the Community*, "because there are multiple foci for decision making, . . . resulting in duplication in some services and gaps in others."[13] In many instances the case manager works with the client and the employer to assist in a timely return to work. The case manager strives to increase client satisfaction through achieving the maximum level of wellness.

The Population Served by Case Management

Case management evolved as a response to the rising cost of health care. A very small percentage of the population uses the majority of health care dollars. About 3 percent of the population uses 40 percent of available health care dollars for the care of catastrophic illness or injury. Seventeen percent of the population uses another 40 percent for chronic illness. The remaining 20 percent of health care dollars is used to treat the remaining 80 percent of the population.[14] Until recently case management services focused on the 20 percent that used 80 percent of the health care dollars. These 20 percent included the elderly and the catastrophically ill or injured. With the rapid changes in health care, and increasing emphasis on prevention, the population benefiting from case management services continues to grow. Today, case management is used for the chronically ill and the well-but-at-risk as well as the catastrophically ill and injured.

Where Case Management is Practiced

Case managers work in various settings. They can be found in the acute care setting, in rehabilitation facilities, in subacute facilities, in community-based programs, in home care, and in insurance companies. In addition, case managers may be independent, on-site representatives of insurance companies. The nurse case manager works collaboratively with the client, family members, significant others, and all members of the interdisciplinary health care team.

THE BEGINNING

Although not a panacea for all that ails the health care system, nursing case management does provide a process for obtaining successful outcomes in a cost-effective, time-efficient manner. During this era of rapid transformation, case management continues to grow and become a more powerful force in creating positive change.

Health care is moving toward primary prevention, and roles for nurses are extending away from acute care settings. The system's demands for economy and efficiency are creating opportunities for nurses to be more autonomous yet simultaneously are generating increasing tension among nurses. A thorough understanding of both the principles and practices of nursing case management will prepare you specifically for this evolving role.

References

1. US Health Care Financing Administration. (1994/Fall). *Health care financing review.* [on-line]
2. Tyson, L. (1993/Oct.6). *The costs of failing to reform health care.* Washington, DC: Council of Economic Advisors. p. 3.
3. Clark, M. (1996). *Nursing in the community.* (2d ed.). Stamford, CT: Appleton & Lange. p. 34.
4. Potter, P., & Perry, A. (1993). *Fundamentals of nursing concepts, process and practice.* (3d ed.). St. Louis: Mosby-Year Book. p. 147.
5. Medical case management a critical factor in health reform. (1995/Nov. 7). Hanover, MD: ICMA [fax transmission].
6. *CCM certification guide.* (1993). Rolling Meadows, IL: CIRSC. Flyleaf.
7. Samrow, S. (1995/Nov.12). Telephone conference.
8. Association of Rehabilitation Nurses. (1995). *The rehabilitation nurse case manager role description.* Skokie, IL.
9. Bower, K. (1992). *Case management by nurses.* Washington, DC: American Nurses Publishing. pp. 7–8.
10. Boling, J. (1996/Oct.). From the field: definitions of case management. *The Case Manager.* 1(3), 35.

11.   Bower, K. (1992). *Case management by nurses*. Washington, DC: American Nurses Publishing. pp. 21–22.

12.   Smith, D. (1995/Oct.). Standards of practice for case management. The importance of practice standards. *The Journal of Care Management*. 1(3), 6.

13.   Clark, M. (1996). *Nursing in the community*. (2d ed.). Stamford, CT: Appleton & Lange. p. 34.

14.   Russell-Babbin, K. (speaker). (1994). Case management: An overview. Villanova, PA: Villanova University.

The Genesis of 2
Case Management

The prolif-
eration of case management throughout all sectors of the health care
delivery system is a relatively recent phenomenon. Case management evolved in response to sky-rocketing health care costs which
have been driven by changes in health care financing and legislation,
technology, and social trends. A brief review of health care history
will explain how and why costs escalated so rapidly.

Upon completion of the chapter you will be able to answer
the following questions:

1. How did the advent of third-party payment for health care
    contribute to the inflation in health care costs?
2. What was the influence of Medicare and Medicaid on health
    care costs?
3. Why has technology been a powerful force in altering
    expectations about health care delivery and associated
    costs?
4. How do the changing demographic characteristics of the
    U.S. population affect health care?

ECONOMIC INFLUENCES

Prior to the 1930s, most health care was paid for by the consumer of care directly to the provider (physician or hospital). This is a two-party payer system; although still in effect today, this system accounts for a relatively small percentage of health care dollars. In the 1930s, private health insurance, a third-party payer system, entered the scene to become the primary mechanism for payment. Following the Great Depression, fewer people were able to afford care, and hospitals and physicians responded by developing prepaid health insurance. This was the beginning of major third-party reimbursement through Blue Cross (to pay hospital expenses) and Blue Shield (to pay physician expenses). People bought insurance to cover health care expenses so that they would no longer have to pay for major expenses "out-of-pocket." Following the success of the Blue Cross and Blue Shield plans, numerous other commercial insurance programs started selling similar policies. As a result, many people now had a mechanism to pay for "catastrophic" or high-end costs associated with hospitalization while they continued to pay for relatively small bills using personal resources.

The Effects of World War II

In the late 1940s, veterans who served in World War II had become accustomed to high-quality care for themselves and their families. Following the war their needs continued to place a strain on health care financing. As veterans entered the work force, numerous employers made health insurance available as an employment bene-fit—many workers preferred this system to salary increases because the benefit had become tax exempt following legislation in 1954.

Thus the stage was set to include a mechanism of payment for health care (health insurance) with virtually no controls or even awareness by consumers as to what such services were costing. Providers of service (primarily hospitals, physicians, and suppliers of equipment, pharmaceuticals, and so on) charged whatever fees they deemed appropriate, and consumers of services merely passed the bills on to the insurance companies for payment. Consumers paid only relatively small bills out-of-pocket, so there was minimal concern or even awareness regarding what was being charged for service. Most insurance policies were purchased by employers and offered as an employee benefit, and this further insulated employees from awareness of any changes in the costs of health care and related increases in the costs of health insurance.

The approach taken by most insurance companies in paying for claims fueled increases in costs. The majority of health insurance policies paid for the "full and reasonable cost" of whatever care was deemed "necessary" by the provider. Claims were paid retrospectively—that is, after the service had been rendered. Thus, providers of care could charge whatever the market would bear as the average patient would not feel the personal effect of charges and providers could obtain substantial profits. In many instances, high charges on those who had insurance coverage was used as a mechanism for providers (physicians and hospitals) to be able to offer care to people who had neither insurance nor personal resources to pay for services (known as *cost-shifting*). Regardless of the provider motivation that propelled ever increasing charges, and because retrospective reimbursement paid in relation to what was charged, an inflationary pattern became established.

Medicare and Medicaid

In 1965, the federally funded Medicare program was established to provide health insurance for the aged and some chronically ill persons. Medicare covers a wide range of services which includes hospitalization, care in skilled nursing facilities, home health care, hospice, physician's services, and a range of outpatient services. By 1991, 30.5 million persons over age 65 and 3.25 million persons with disabilities were receiving benefits paid for by Medicare.[1] By 1994, this had increased to 36 million people, which is more than 10 percent of our total population.[2] Providing for these services has had a profound economic effect on the U.S. economy. Whereas the budget for Medicare was $4.7 billion in 1967, by 1992 it had increased 2800 percent to $132 billion.[3] If there are no changes in the current structure of Medicare, it is projected that the expenditures will exceed $327 billion by the year 2000.[4] Medicaid, a grant program funded by both the federal and state governments, was also established in 1965. The purpose was to provide financial access to health care for the "medically indigent." Although some people automatically qualify for Medicaid coverage due to federal requirements of the program, for the most part each state defines income qualifications as well as optional services to be covered. During the 1970s and 1980s, the number of Medicaid beneficiaries remained relatively stable at approximately 21.5 million. However, the recession of the early 1990s resulted in a substantial increase in the number of people eligible for Medicaid. By 1991, there were 27 million enrolled in the program, and this number is likely to grow. In 1968, the combined expense of Medicaid to the state and federal government was approximately $3.45 billion; it is anticipated that the cost will reach $158 billion in 1996.[5] Whereas Medicare and Medicaid have served recipients well by ensuring access to health care they might otherwise be denied, it has also greatly added to the cost of delivering services. There have been few restrictions on how much or how frequently a person could have service, and this helped to fuel the rapid increase in health care expenditure.

THE INFLUENCE OF LEGISLATION

As early as 1946, legislation was enacted that would, over time, have a major impact on escalating health care costs. The *Hospital and Construction Act of 1946* (commonly known as the *Hill-Burton Act*), provided federal matching grant funds for construction and expansion of health care facilities. Over the years the funding was renewed several times, and the legislation did support funding for more than 20 percent of the new hospital beds built from 1946 to

1966. Although the intent of the bill was to provide funding for needed beds, political pressure was more powerful than rational planning, and a substantial oversupply of beds was created. The financial pressure to keep these beds full, in conjunction with an as yet financially unregulated health care delivery system, was a significant force in driving up the cost of health care.

In 1965, Medicare was enacted as Title XVIII of the *Social Security Act*. Although there was powerful support to provide health insurance coverage to a sector of the population considered vulnerable, over time the program costs rose prohibitively and threatened its very survival. The *Omnibus Budget Reconciliation Act of 1981* (OBRA–P.L. 97-35) initiated substantial budget cuts which reduced funding of Medicare. By 1982, the *Tax Equity and Fiscal Responsibility Act* (TEFRA–P.L. 97-248) required development of prospective payment systems in an effort to regain control over costs. This was followed by the *Social Security Amendments of 1983* (P.L. 98-21), also referred to as the "DRG law," which established the use of prospective payment based on diagnosis related groups (DRGs). In this model, each patient who is admitted to a hospital is assigned a pretreatment diagnosis, and it is this diagnosis, in combination with whether there are surgery and any comorbidities, which determines exactly what the hospital will receive as reimbursement for care. From 1983 on, continued efforts have been directed at reducing the rate of inflation in both Medicare and Medicaid expenses with rather disappointing results.

THE EFFECT OF TECHNOLOGY

Whereas advances in medical technology have had a positive impact on both quality of life and life expectancy, these improvements have created an enormous drain on financial resources. Advances in diagnostic techniques such as magnetic resonance imaging (MRI) and computerized tomography (CT), complex long-term treatments such as maintaining ventilator-dependent clients at home, and providing life-sustaining treatment for neonates born as early as 23 to

24 weeks gestation has stretched cure and care far beyond anything envisioned even a decade ago.

Even less exotic technological improvements such as ultrasound evaluation of the fetus in utero or use of radioactive isotopes in a thallium stress test to evaluate cardiac disease have become so commonplace that consumers not only ask for but often demand the use of technology. Historically, physicians have had relatively few guidelines regarding diagnostic protocols, and so their use proliferated. This trend has been further supported by physician concern over increasing the potential for malpractice suits because a diagnosis that could have been made with the technology was missed without its use.

A contributing factor to technological proliferation is our massive industrial complex in pharmaceuticals and medical devices. The United States is the world leader in this area and on the cutting edge of most scientific developments. However, such research carries an expensive price tag. Businesses which allocate substantial resources to the development of new drugs and medical products do so with the knowledge and expectation that capital invested will be made back in profits. Thus, although the actual production cost of a new drug could be as little as $1 per dose, to regain the investment in research and development and marketing and still make a profit, the manufacturer might have to charge as much as $5.

Over the past 25 years, the combination of advances in medical diagnosis with those in treatment, many of which have been facilitated by newly developed technology, has created dramatic changes in how we experience health and illness. Although most would probably concur that they have benefited from the development of medical technology, they would also have to acknowledge that it has carried a robust price tag.

CHANGING MORBIDITY PATTERNS

Developments in medical science generated great advances in the diagnosis and treatment of diseases that had been major threats to health and well-being at the beginning of the twentieth century. Antibiotics led to the ability to control infectious diseases; greater knowledge supported advances in the care of pregnant women and neonates; vaccines were developed that could prevent dread diseases such as polio; and technology such as kidney dialysis made it possible to survive, and even work, while in complete kidney shutdown.

Unfortunately, these substantial gains have come to be more than offset by a host of health problems that may be influenced by lifestyle. AIDS, a disease which did not even exist prior to the 1980s, has become one of the major sources of disability and death in our population and has the potential of reaching epidemic proportions. Tuberculosis, once considered cured by newly developed drugs, has now emerged in a frightening drug-resistant form. Substance abuse is rampant, and it is estimated that as many as 375,000 babies are born each year to addicted mothers. Depression, suicide, and violence have become so pervasive that it is difficult to even know where to start to tackle these problems.

We have become a society of "couch potatoes"—overweight, sedentary, feeling stressed, and overburdened. These are all factors that place many at risk for related illnesses. When we add to this numerous environmental pollutants, smoking, unemployment, underemployment, violence, and poverty, we recognize the converging risk factors for a range of morbidities. As a result, when medical science has given us the potential to be the healthiest ever possible, some lifestyle choices have generated a dismal picture of our well-being.

SOCIAL TRENDS

The characteristics of the U.S. population have been changing in terms of age distribution, morbidity patterns, and lifestyles. Of the 250 million people reported in the 1990 U.S. census, the median age had increased from 30.0 years in 1980 to the current 33.1 years. Almost thirteen percent of the population is over age 65, and it is expected that the year 2000 will see approximately 36 million Americans over age 65. The fastest growing segment of the population is the "very old" or people over age 85.[6] As the population ages, its consumption of health care dollars increases. Not only are there more episodic illness events, but also more people live with multiple chronic illnesses.

Family structures have also been changing. There are fewer nuclear families, and the tendency for families to remain in a geographic area has been replaced by a trend to move often to either retain employment or seek new employment. Many aging people no longer can count on the presence or support of their children and family members to provide care during episodic or chronic illness. Families who often are having difficulty maintaining their own integrity have little ability to contribute to the care of another family member. This results in increased demand for community-based services to provide care that traditionally was thought to be a family responsibility. And such care must be paid for.

At the other end of the age spectrum, the rate of teenage pregnancy has escalated to the degree that by 1990, teenage birth rates have exceeded those in most of the industrially developed world. Teenage pregnancies are generally considered high-risk, and their newborns have a disproportionate incidence of problems with physical health, social and emotional development, and cognitive development. This creates significant financial burden on society to meet the health care needs of at-risk teenagers and their babies.

CONCLUSION

Economics, legislation, technology, morbidity patterns, and social trends have all contributed in some way to the uncontrolled growth of health care costs. Any single element operating alone would probably not have had the power to create a change of such magnitude. However, the effect of these factors coming together in a relatively short period created a scenario ready for change. It was in this environment that "external" case management emerged in the 1970s as insurance companies sought a mechanism to ensure the best utilization and client outcomes for the dollars they spent in reimbursement. By the 1980s, acute care facilities were feeling the financial impact of curtailed revenue that resulted from a prospective reimbursement system. A natural outcome was the development of "internal" case management, and the stage was set for continued development of this role across the continuum of care in every type of health care facility.

Chapter Highlights

* The model of traditional indemnity insurance fostered relatively uncontrolled growth in both the delivery and cost of health care services.

* In 1965, federally funded Medicare and Medicaid programs extended health insurance to many previously uninsured people. These programs continued the acceleration of health care inflation.

* Technology has made marked advances in the diagnosis and treatment of a wide range of problems. The development and use of technology has been prohibitively expensive.

* Changing lifestyles and sociodemographic trends have contributed to the development of more chronic illness that is costly to treat. As our population ages, more health care dollars are being consumed than at any time in the past.

* Case management originated in the 1970s in the insurance industry and was further developed in acute care hospitals in the 1980s. At this time, case management is found in virtually every sector of the health care delivery system.

1. U.S. Department of Commerce. (1993). *Statistical abstract of the United States, 1993.* [on-line].
2. *Health: United States, 1993.* (1994). DHHS Pub No (PHS) 94-1232. [on-line].
3. Smith, C., & Maurer, F. (1995). *Community health nursing: Theory and practice.* Philadelphia, PA: W.B. Saunders Co. p. 20.
4. Health Insurance Association of America. (1995). *Source book of health insurance data: 1994.* Washington, DC: p. 65.
5. Congressional Budget Office (1992/Oct.). *Economic implications of rising health care costs.* [on-line].
6. *The world almanac and book of facts.* (1994). Mahwah, NJ: Funk and Wagnalls. pp. 358–422.

The Relationship of 3
Insurance Coverage
and Case
Management

For case managers to broker services effectively for clients across the health care continuum, they must understand the variety of mechanisms that currently exist to pay for health care services. This chapter explores the types of health insurance currently available to pay for health care.

Upon completion of this chapter, you will be able to answer the following questions:

1. What are the differences among the types of group health insurance plans?
2. What is the financial impact of managed care plans on the consumer as well as on the provider?
3. What is the coverage generally provided by Medicare, Medicaid, motor vehicle insurance, and workers' compensation insurance?
4. How does the type of insurance coverage influence the role of the case manager?

The following are some key words used in this chapter:

Capitation: A method of payment to providers for health care services rendered. The payment is negotiated and paid on a fixed (per capita or per head) amount for each person receiving care regardless of the frequency or type of service given. The goal of capitation is to reduce health care expenses by encouraging more conservative health care delivery.

Current procedural terminology (CPT) code: A systematic listing of procedures and services performed by physicians. Each specific procedure or service has an assigned five-digit code. The codes provide a uniform language that accurately describes medical, surgical, and diagnostic procedures. The codes are needed to report services rendered to insurance carriers.

Health maintenance organization (HMO): This organization of doctors, hospitals, and other allied health professionals provides comprehensive service, usually focusing on primary prevention, to an enrolled population for a fixed, predetermined fee. The monthly fee remains the same regardless of the types or levels of services provided. Its physicians are either employed by the HMO or under contract with the HMO (in which case the physician provides service in a private office).

International classification of diseases, clinical modification (ICD-9-CM): A statistical classification system that organizes diseases and injuries into groups according to standardized criteria. Each diagnosis is assigned a three-, four-, or five-digit code number. The codes are used by insurance carriers to reimburse providers. (Note: There is a major difference between ICD and CPT codes. The ICD code is assigned to a *disease* and the CPT code designates a *procedure*).

Indemnity insurance: Traditional health insurance that provides benefits when the eligible insured person incurs expenses for the treatment of an illness or accident. Also called "fee for service."

Managed care: A range of techniques designed to deliver quality health care services to the consumer while minimizing the costs to the health care provider or to the third-party payer.

Point-of-service program (POS): A type of managed care program in which the individual may seek health care service from a provider either within or outside the insurance network. Individuals have the lowest out-of-pocket expenses if they first seek care from a participating primary care provider and have proper authorization prior to seeing a specialist.

Preferred provider organization (PPO): A network of health care providers who have contracted to provide designated professional services to insured individuals at a discounted fee.

Primary care provider (PCP): Also referred to as *primary care manager*, the health care professional, most often a physician, who is responsible for care management of insured individuals. This professional provides primary care services to patients and is responsible for authorizing referrals to more specialized physicians for specialist care.

Provider: A health care professional who is licensed to deliver a specific type of service to the client. Includes physicians, nurses, therapists, pharmacists, vendors of durable medical equipment, laboratories, imaging services, and so on.

FINANCING HEALTH CARE

Health care is a service or commodity which must be paid for by the care recipient just as any other service or commodity must be. At the present time, a variety of health insurance plans provide payment for health care expenses. In the private sector, over 1500 commercial insurance companies provide coverage to those who purchase policies. Such group health insurance (GHI) policies may be purchased by individuals, families, or employers who pay some portion of the cost of insurance (premium) as a fringe benefit of employment. In some large businesses, employers may choose to "self-insure," which means that they budget a certain amount to cover the health care expenses of employees and avoid paying an insurance carrier premiums to assume the risk of coverage. Many companies who are self-insured hire outside firms to maintain all records regarding the people covered by the insurance plan. These outside firms, called *third-party administrators* (TPAs) may also be responsible for the actual disbursement of funds to pay the claims.

A Brief History of Insurance

Health insurance began in the mid-1800s when private insurance companies began writing policies that would provide benefits to pay the treatment costs for a limited number of diseases. These plans "indemnified" (i.e., compensated for expenses incurred) the individual who purchased the policy. A potential flaw in this system was that the provider of health care had to be paid for services by the recipient, and many providers had difficulty collecting the fees due them.

This method was altered when, in 1929, a group of teachers in Texas contracted with Baylor Hospital to provide room, board, and ancillary services at a predetermined cost per month.[1] This type of contract was the precursor of what became known as Blue Cross plans. These plans were well received by hospitals, which favored the plans because the payment for services rendered went directly to the hospital. Shortly thereafter, similar plans were developed by physicians to cover the costs of medical services— these plans became known as Blue Shield.

The trend of increasing health insurance coverage for the working population was strengthened during World War II. During that period there were wage freezes, and group health insurance was offered as a means of enhancing employees benefits. In industries with collective bargaining contracts, health insurance quickly became a covered (and negotiated) benefit.

Through the 1950s and 1960s, the country experienced a period of rapid economic expansion and population growth. In the field of medicine, numerous technical advancements occurred, and many new diagnostic and treatment options became available. The health insurance policies available up to that time had been designed primarily to pay for limited hospital and physician expenses; they were insufficient for the newly expanding scope of services. The health insurance industry began to offer a new type of coverage that allowed for services which were broader, potentially more expensive, and of longer duration. This was the birth of major medical insurance. The intent of this insurance was to protect insured individuals from "catastrophic" expenses—those that could not be afforded by most people in society. It was not intended that health insurance be the vehicle for payment of almost all or even all expenses, although, over time, this expectation has become the norm.

Just as insurance is intended to protect people from catastrophic expenses, insurance companies also have a mechanism to protect them from very expensive claims. These insurance carriers purchase a "reinsurance policy" which transfers some of the economic cost to yet another insurance company for a set premium.

Indemnity Insurance

Traditionally, the health insurance available has been of the "indemnity" or "fee-for-service" type. Any insurance policy specifies the terms and conditions that apply, including:

- The types of services covered
- The types of providers whose services will be paid
- The deductible (number of dollars the person must spend out-of-pocket before the insurance begins to cover expenses)
- The copay or coinsurance (either a fixed dollar amount the person pays per encounter or office visit or the percentage of the usual, customary, and reasonable fee for which the individual is responsible)
- The stop-loss level (the figure at which the insurance will pay 100 percent of the costs incurred)
- The maximum the policy will pay (usually expressed as a dollar amount over a period of time)

Traditional indemnity insurance offers the maximum flexibility to the consumer; there are relatively few restrictions as to when, where, or from whom the health care is accessed or purchased. A "typical" indemnity policy is likely to cover almost any service deemed medically necessary by a licensed physician. The covered individual often spends from $200 to $1000 or more out-of-pocket (the annual deductible) before the insurance starts to cover expenses. After the deductible is met, the client still may pay 20 cents of each dollar of health care expenses (20 percent coinsurance, or whatever percentage is specified by the policy) until the stop-loss level is reached. This might be at $2500, $5000, or even $10,000, depending on the specific policy.

Although indemnity insurance is generally favored by most consumers because of the freedom of choice allowed, it now is the most expensive coverage to purchase. These policies carry the highest premiums and the largest out-of-pocket expenses of all types of health insurance because of several converging factors. The insurance company pays the provider on a retrospective basis—that is, it reimburses for service after the service has been provided. The fee charged by the provider is not controlled, and the insurance company pays at a fixed percentage of what is defined as the *UCR*, that is, the "usual, customary and reasonable" fee for a particular service (by CPT code and ICD9 diagnosis) in a given geographic area (often defined by zip code). In addition, the rapid development of sophisticated high-tech diagnostic and treatment approaches has generated increased demand for use by both providers and consumers. Technology has significantly increased the cost of care. Retrospective payment has contributed to the inflation in health care costs and provides no incentive to providers or consumers to plan for more efficient use of health care services.[2]

EVOLUTION OF MANAGED CARE

In an effort to control skyrocketing health care costs, many insurance companies worked aggressively in the 1980s to develop a model of health insurance that would control and balance the cost of health care while maintaining quality. The result has been the evolution of systems of managed care which range from the least restrictive preferred provider organization to the most highly controlled health maintenance organization. An important aspect of the managed care approach is that the providers of care share some of the financial risk that the insurance company has traditionally carried alone, thus motivating providers to practice in a cost-efficient manner. Using a combination of factors, health insurance companies are currently writing policies in a vast number of ways. However, for our purposes, it is most important to understand the major concepts of how managed care systems organize to deliver care and at the same time control costs.

The Preferred Provider Organization

The least intrusive approach in terms of how "controlled" access to care becomes is the PPO. In a PPO, a variety of health care providers such as physicians, therapists, nursing agencies, diagnostic facilities, and equipment vendors agree to discount their usual fees and provide services to the consumer for a previously negotiated price. The consumer who seeks care from providers within the PPO will have the lowest personal cost. A consumer wishing to seek care from a provider not in the PPO is likely to incur a substantially larger noncovered expense. In the event that the individual wishes to seek services of a specialist, an appointment can be made without first consulting the primary care physician.

Preferred provider organizations are somewhat effective in cost containment because the provider fees are discounted to the insurance company, and there is some incentive for the provider of service to keep operating costs as low as possible. However, some inflationary pressure present in traditional indemnity coverage spills over into PPOs as there is virtually no restriction on the quantity or frequency of service the consumer can access.

As an example of how a PPO saves money for both the consumer and the insurance company, consider this simple scenario of health care delivery. A young man has a fever of 102° F, a sore throat, and swollen glands. He has been ill for 2 days and shows no signs of improvement. He makes an appointment with his primary care provider who is a family practitioner. The costs incurred under a traditional indemnity plan are as follows:

Office visit (exam)	=	$ 50.00
Rapid strep test	=	25.00 (test is positive for beta hemolytic group A strep)
Treatment	=	10.85 for Amoxicillin 250 mg, 1 cap TID × 10 days
Repeat strep test	=	25.00 (done when treatment is completed)
Total cost:	=	$110.85

Since this is the client's first medical expense of the year, all the $110.85 will have to be paid out-of-pocket but will count toward meeting his insurance deductible should he incur additional expenses this year.

Now consider the same situation if the client is with a PPO. The costs incurred are as follows:

Office visit (exam)	=	$50.00 (Insurance carrier will actually reimburse the MD $38, the negoti- ated rate)
Rapid strep test	=	16.75 (the negotiated rate)
Treatment	=	9.00 (the negotiated rate)
Repeat strep test	=	16.75 (the negotiated rate and done when _____ treatment is complete)
Total cost	=	$92.50

As you can see, the client could save $18.35 for one of the least complex and most common kind of medical service. Likewise, the insurance company also saves if the claim is to be reimbursed. Under indemnity coverage, the carrier would pay 80 percent of $110.85 (or whatever percent is specified by the policy). Under

PPO coverage, the carrier's cost would be 80 percent of $92.50 (or other designated percent) which would save $7.40. Although this particular saving might not seem that large, imagine what it could add up to multiplied by many thousands of subscribers in a PPO and numerous diagnostic and therapeutic procedures that are substantially more expensive! Even for treatment as basic as physical therapy for an injury, if the full fee is $100 per visit and 12 weeks of therapy three times per week has been ordered, the cost will be $3600. The same treatment in a PPO, where the negotiated rate is $75 per visit, would cost $2700. In this case the savings of $900 would be completely realized by the insurance carrier.

Although there is tremendous diversity both in how PPOs organize to provide service and in the nature of the financial relationship between insurer and client, a few operational elements are incorporated almost universally in PPOs. These include:

- Restriction of the number of providers included in the PPO. Sponsoring organizations such as insurers or hospitals will contract with a predetermined number of providers who meet specific criteria in terms of credentials, cost-efficiency, and scope of service.
- Negotiated payments. The providers who join the PPO network have agreed to accept a negotiated level of reimbursement.
- Utilization review (UR). Participating providers agree to abide by the utilization review procedures administered by the PPO. UR is a process which evaluates the appropriateness of services planned (in terms of medical necessity and appropriateness of the level of care) prior to the actual delivery of service. The major goal is to eliminate waste and potential risks to the patient.[3]

The Point-of-Service Plan

A somewhat more restrictive and rapidly growing type of insurance coverage that is designed to include the advantages of indemnity coverage (which allows maximum flexibility) and diminish the disadvantage of uncontrolled cost is the point-of-service plan. In a POS plan, each consumer chooses a PCP from a list of physicians who have contracted with the network or insurance carrier. The PCP acts as "gatekeeper" for all the health care needs of the consumer. The PCP provides referrals to specialty and ancillary services. In most POS plans the PCP has a financial incentive to make referrals judiciously as the PCP may be penalized if the insurance carrier deems that there is a pattern of excessive use of specialty and/or diagnostic services. Should this occur, the insurance carrier can reduce fees that the PCP is eligible to receive (such as an end-of-year monetary bonus for meeting specific performance standards) and can even remove the PCP from the network of providers.

Point-of-service plans reimburse the PCP in one of two ways. Some plans use retrospective reimbursement for services rendered according to a previously negotiated fee schedule similar to the reimbursement in a PPO system. Other plans use prospective reimbursement through a system of capitation. Capitation is discussed later in this chapter in the section on HMOs.

Individuals having POS insurance tend to gain financially because there are relatively few out-of-pocket expenses as long as service is obtained from the PCP. In most cases, a typical office visit to the PCP will require a copay of $5 to $20 with no additional expense. If specialist services are needed, as long as the individual obtains appropriate referral from the PCP to a specialist within the network, only a copay will be required. Clients who wish to have complete freedom of choice in accessing service can opt to go out of the network. This generally entails higher out-of-pocket expense as well as the possibility that some services will not be covered (most commonly, those geared toward primary prevention).

Point-of-service plans share several common features:

- The use of the PCP as a gatekeeper to control referrals to specialists

- Allowing the individual to use out-of-network providers but at a lower benefit level (i.e., greater out-of-pocket expense)
- Allowing the individual to seek care in or out of the network at each "point of service" or each time care is sought.[4]

Point-of-service plans have been gaining in popularity. In 1990 POS plans accounted for only 2 percent of the enrollment in health care plans, but by 1993 the figure had increased to 9 percent. Current projections are that by the end of 1996 POS plans will account for 15 percent of all enrollment in private health care plans.[5]

The Health Maintenance Organization

The most restrictive and, many believe, the most cost-efficient model for financing health care is the health maintenance organization. This type of health care delivery system, created by the Health Maintenance Organization Act of 1973, stipulates that federally designated HMOs must meet four criteria: (1) provision of an organized system of health care in a particular geographic area, (2) a predetermined set of services for health maintenance and treatment, (3) voluntary enrollment, and (4) rates of service comparable to those for similar services in the geographic area.[6]

The cost efficiency of HMOs is a direct outcome of the method of paying for care and controls placed on how health care service is accessed. Most HMOs have a per capita prospective reimbursement system for providers. The health care provider agrees that for a predetermined fee per person per year, the provider will make available all covered services needed. This model emphasizes health promotion and disease prevention: If the clients are healthy, high-cost medical procedures and, most notably, hospital admissions are reduced. Because HMOs operate on a fixed budget, providers must be especially sensitive to consumer utilization patterns.

Many consumers, especially healthy adults, find that HMOs are a very satisfactory form of health insurance. Although the consumer is restricted to receiving care only from a designated primary care provider (who is usually chosen by the consumer from a network), the out-of-pocket expenses are minimal. There usually is no deductible to be met before the HMO pays for service, and for most consumers the only personal expense is a copayment for each physician visit (generally $2 to $20, depending on the specifics of the contract). The consumer rarely has to pay any of the cost of diagnostic procedures or a range of therapeutic interventions. Dissatisfaction for individuals enrolled in HMOs usually stems from the restrictions the HMO mandates. For example, an individual who believes specialty care is required must first get it authorized by the primary care provider. Primary care providers tend to be very conservative in referring a client for specialist services, and most of the care is delivered by generalists in HMOs. Emergency room visits are often not reimbursed if the presenting problem does not lead to hospital admission.

Much of the cost savings achieved by HMOs is attributed to the reduction of costly hospitalization and a shift to less expensive ambulatory care services. In addition, a practice style is imposed on the primary care provider. Because the provider is compensated at a fixed dollar amount per individual per year regardless of the frequency or scope of service actually rendered, through capitation, there is incentive both to limit the number of visits the individual has per year and to restrict the types of diagnostic and therapeutic procedures. There is a growing concern that HMOs have great potential for overly restricting access to care, especially for the elderly and for persons with chronic conditions. If HMO delivery trends continue, the result is likely to be a reduction in quality of care with the potential for less satisfactory client outcomes.[7]

Despite the concerns expressed by many health care professionals, membership in HMOs has grown rapidly from approximately 3 million subscribers in 1970 to 18.9 million in 1985. Since then, enrollment has increased to more than 45 million.[8] It is likely that this trend will continue for some time, especially in light of the current economic forces influencing health care.

PUBLICLY FUNDED INSURANCE

Thus far the discussion has focused on third-party payment for health care expenses in the private sector through group health insurance. However, since 1965, when federal legislation created Medicare and Medicaid, the federal and state governments have become major players as third-party payers through publicly funded health insurance. Access to health care services for the elderly has been greatly expanded through Medicare. Whereas only half of the elderly had any health insurance prior to 1965, today this is the only age group in the United States that has universal coverage (although there are limitations on types of services covered). The medically indigent, although better protected since the initiation of Medicaid, still tend to experience serious limitations in accessing many types of health care services. Because there is extensive debate over these programs and proposed legislation that could substantively alter the funding, the nature of the publicly funded programs and scope of services provided may be markedly different in the future.

The following describes publicly funded programs as they exist in 1996.

Medicare

Medicare is a federally funded insurance program created by Title XIX of the Social Security Act. Medicare has two distinct coverage components—Part A, the Hospital Insurance Program, and Part B, the Supplemental Medical Insurance Program. All people 65 years and older who are eligible for Social Security benefits are eligible for Medicare. Some individuals qualify for Medicare at a younger age due to disability (which establishes eligibility for Social Security Disability) or due to permanent kidney failure, which requires dialysis. Part A coverage is funded by Social Security taxes and is provided to all eligible individuals at no personal expense. Part B coverage is optional, and individuals who select this coverage pay a monthly premium (similar to private health insurance although less expensive).

Medicare Part A covers hospital care and a range of related services as follows:

- Semiprivate room, lab tests, x-rays, medications, nursing services, operating room (OR), recovery room (RR). Client has a deductible of $716 per benefit period and varying copays for days 61 to 150 of each admission.
- Skilled nursing facility (SNF) or extended care facility (ECF): semiprivate room, skilled nursing and rehabilitative services, medications, supplies. Client has no deductible but has a copay of $89.50 per day for days 21 to 100. Client can be admitted to a SNF only following a minimum of a 3-day stay in an acute care facility.
- Home health care: individual must be homebound, require intermittent (as opposed to intensive) skilled nursing care or skilled rehabilitation therapies. The plan of care must be ordered and periodically reviewed by a physician. Care must be obtained from a Medicare-certified agency. Client has no deductible but has a copay of 20 percent for durable medical equipment (DME), which includes items such as wheelchairs, nebulizers, etc.
- Hospice care: individual must be judged terminally ill by the treating physician. Client has no deductible but has a copay of 20 percent for DME and $5 or 5 percent of the cost of drugs for pain relief.[9]

Medicare Part B is a supplemental insurance policy that covers services of physicians, other health care providers such as physical and occupational therapists, outpatient clinic and emergency room services, laboratory and diagnostic services, durable medical equipment, and a limited range of medications (primarily IV medications to be administered to clients at home). Under Part B, the individual pays an annual deductible of $100 and is responsible for a 20 percent copay for most services. The current cost of the Medicare Part B premium is $46.10 per month per individual.

Although Medicare has successfully provided health insurance to a sizable component of the population, the system is fraught with problems. The increasing cost of providing the coverage has generated higher premiums for Part B and higher deductibles for Part A. Medicare does not cover many of the services most required by the population, such as prescription drugs to manage chronic illnesses, primary prevention services, and supportive (custodial) care to maintain people in the home environment.

Medicaid

Medicaid is a national program also established by Title XIX of the Social Security Act. The program, a part of the federal and state welfare system, provides access to health care by people deemed "categorically needy" or "medically needy." *Categorically needy* includes people who are eligible for Aid to Families with Dependent Children (AFDC) or Supplemental Security Income (SSI). The *medically needy* includes people who are financially able to meet their basic needs but have inadequate resources to pay for health care needs.

The services and eligibility for Medicaid vary from state to state. However, under the provision of the initial legislation, all Medicaid programs are required to provide a set of federally mandated services. The federally mandated services include:

- Hospital inpatient care and outpatient services
- Skilled nursing care
- Physician services
- Home health care
- Family planning services
- Early and periodic screening, diagnosis and treatment for children under age 21 (EPSDT)[10]

Medicaid is funded by the general tax revenues of the federal and state governments. The people covered by Medicaid have no out-of-pocket expense for the coverage. Until recently, Medicaid generally reimbursed providers on a fee-for-service basis and hospitals on a per diem basis. However, as the cost of the program has escalated, many states have reduced either the level and scope of services available or the number of people eligible for Medicaid. Furthermore, reduction of the reimbursement to providers for some services has created shortages of providers in parts of the country.

Government-funded insurance has experienced the same escalating costs as the private insurance industry. The same forces—an aging population; medical care driven by costly technology; chronic diseases; health problems resulting from poverty, ignorance, and violence; and changing epidemiology with diseases such as AIDS—affect the system regardless of who is paying the bill. For this reason, the government insurance plans have initiated cost-containment strategies that rely heavily on the use of managed care, using strategies similar to the methods employed in the private sector.

Despite the effort to develop insurance plans designed to control costs while maintaining quality care, the cost of health care in the United States has continued to grow at an alarming rate. Health care in 1965, which accounted for 5.0 percent of the gross domestic product (GDP), represented a per capita expense of $204 or a total of $41.6 billion. By 1993, this had increased to 13.9 percent of the GDP or $3299 per person with a total spending of $884.2 billion.[11] Assuming no major reform of the health care delivery system, it is estimated that by the year 2000 health care spending will account for 18 percent of the GDP![12]

HOW INSURANCE INFLUENCES
THE ROLE OF THE CASE MANAGER

Nurse case managers can play an important part in the care of the individual who has experienced catastrophic illness or injury or chronic illness. Each insurer has independent criteria regarding the circumstances and diagnoses for which case management is to be undertaken. However, the universal goal is to maximize the client's outcomes in the most cost-effective way. For the most part, individuals with the following diagnoses are likely candidates for case management:

- High-risk antepartal women (e.g., diabetics, substance abusers)
- High-risk neonates (e.g., those with congenital anomalies, very low birth weight)
- Major chronic illnesses (e.g., AIDS, degenerative neuromuscular conditions, Alzheimer's disease, diabetes mellitus with complications)
- Cancer (end-stage disease with prognosis of less than 6 months' life expectancy)
- Head trauma and spinal cord injuries
- Any illness or injury which will require substantial treatment and technology after discharge from the hospital (ventilator dependence, IV therapy, TPN)

The nurse case manager is responsible for developing a plan of care that is appropriate, high-quality, and cost-effective. How important the specific details of the client's insurance coverage are vary depending on the setting. In all situations, the case manager should understand the major coverage components available to the client for planning purposes. These include: What types of services are covered? For how long will the insurance carrier pay for service? Are there any restrictions placed so that only specific providers can be used for care and equipment? Is there a maximum dollar amount the insurer will pay per illness or in a given period of time? The plan of care which is developed must be acceptable to the client but must also be authorized by the insurance carrier who ultimately "pays the bill." Given the real world constraints on resources, the nurse case manager is always trying to "stretch" dollars—to have the client achieve the best outcome possible before benefits are exhausted. This is especially significant when working with individuals predicted to have high-end treatment costs. For example, the lifetime medical treatment costs alone for an individual with congenital rubella syndrome may be around $354,000 and for an individual with quadriplegia from a spinal cord injury they are $570,000.[13] It must be noted that these are the costs for *medical treatment* only and do not include the expenses of special education, vocational rehabilitation, home modification, and so on.

The type of insurance coverage available to your clients can affect them greatly. What the client desires in terms of treatment may or may not be reimbursable by the insurance carrier. As more people become insured by managed care plans, the number and range of options available for diagnosis and treatment are shrinking. For the individual confronting a catastrophic illness or accident, the limits on the potential scope of services reimbursable by the insurance carrier create an additional source of stress and anxiety. The nurse case manager now confronts an individual who must deal not only with the psychosocial impact of serious illness but also with the stress of additional financial concerns. For clients with chronic illness, many similar concerns exist. These clients also fear that health care needs will exceed benefits judged allowable by the insurance carrier. If this occurs, the client with chronic illness, and often deteriorating health status, will have to manage with a decreased level and scope of health care service. The type of group health insurance coverage will greatly influence the type of service, duration of service, and type of facility in which the catastrophically ill, injured, or chronically ill person will receive care.

WORKERS' COMPENSATION INSURANCE AND CASE MANAGEMENT

Many of the clients who receive case management services have experienced injuries or illnesses that are work related. In this situation, the health care expenses are paid for by workers' compensation insurance. This type of program was initiated in 1911 when the industrial boom was in full swing. At that time, following injury, many workers and their families became penniless when the main wage earner was injured on the job. Workers' compensation is the oldest social insurance program in the United States. By 1948, all states had passed this type of legislation.

Workers' compensation is mandated and funded by each state independently. Although the programs vary markedly from state to state, they all provide cash benefits and health care to a worker who suffers a work-related injury or temporary or permanent disability or who dies (in which case the family receives cash benefits). Each state sets a minimum and maximum range for benefits; on the average, workers receive 66 percent of their previous gross salary. The higher the wages earned prior to injury, the greater the loss of income experienced.

Characteristics of the Law

Workers' compensation law is based on a no-fault, limited liability system. This means that the worker is awarded compensation regardless of who is at fault for the occurrence. Employers may choose to purchase the insurance coverage through a private insurance carrier or through the state-operated insurance fund where available, or they may give proof of financial ability to act as self-insurers.

All compensation acts require that an injured worker receives medical care without delay, and there is no limit on the amount of medical care the worker can receive when accidental injury is involved. All states require that the cost of care is covered from the first dollar, so the worker has no out-of-pocket expenses directly related to medical care for work-related injury or illness. The individual's ability to select the health care provider varies. In some states, such as New York, the person may choose any primary care provider. In other states, such as New Jersey, the employer selects the provider who will diagnose and treat the employee. Another variable is the reimbursement to the health care provider. A state either may mandate payment according to the UCR or may utilize a fee schedule which specifies the exact compensation per CPT code (type of service rendered) and ICDM-9 diagnosis. See Table 3-1 for a comparison of group health insurance and workers' compensation insurance.

Workers' compensation statutes are designed to protect both the employee and the employer. There is concern that resources be used wisely and that disputes over degree of injury and continuing disability are resolved. In most states, an independent medical examination (IME) by someone other than the treating physician can be required by the employer. Once the worker is judged able to return to work, the compensation award is usually terminated. In some states workers can receive benefits for only a specific period of time or for a specific dollar amount even if there is permanent disability.

Table 3-1. Group Health Insurance and Workers' Compensation Insurance

Characteristic	Group Health Insurance	Workers' Compensation
Definition	Broad-coverage insurance purchased by an individual, family or employer	A social contract between employer & employee that provides a no-fault source of insurance to pay for injuries and illnesses that occur at work
Scope of coverage	Usually includes a waiting period before coverage is active, and pre-existing conditions are often excluded. Coverage applies regardless of where or how the injury/ illness occurred. Coverage is "treatment"-based and pays for treatment only as long as policy is in effect. If employee changes jobs there may be a lapse in coverage. Many categories of workers (e.g., part-time, seasonal) are not covered.	Virtually all workers are covered (full-time, part-time, temporary) with only a few categories excluded. Coverage begins on the first day of work. Coverage based on an "occurrence" basis. Once the work-related illness or injury has occurred, the insurance coverage continues even if the worker changes jobs or retires.

Mandatory or voluntary	Voluntary for the employer and usually offered as a fringe benefit of employment. Employer determines type of policy to purchase as well as the level of benefits. No regulatory agency supervision.	Mandatory–each state dictates the type of benefits that must be provided to employees. Employer has option to purchase coverage or self-insure.
Benefits	Pays for medical treatment services as specified by the insurance contract. Policies usually have either a yearly maximum and/or lifetime maximum in dollar amount. Does not include vocational rehab services, disability payments, or death benefits.	Differ among states but generally cover all reasonably required medical services to cure or relieve the effects of injury or illness. No dollar maximum on services provided as long as medically necessary. Includes vocational rehab services, a wage-replacement component for the period the employee is unable to work, and payment for permanent impairment as well as payment in the case of employee death.
Cost of policy	Costs determined by insurance carrier with minimal government regulation on premiums. Employees usually share a portion of the cost through copays, deductibles and possibly by paying a portion of the monthly premium.	Costs are regulated by the state's insurance commission. Costs of premiums are the responsibility of the employer alone, and there are no contributions by the employee.

Difficulties Encountered with Workers' Compensation

Workers' compensation insurance has become a subject of great concern to employers, legislators, and health care providers because it remains one of the few insurance programs with virtually no cost-containment methods. In addition, weaknesses in the system have allowed fraud to become a substantial issue. Many workers malinger, and a recent survey indicates that there is a perception that knowing cooperation between injured workers and lawyers, doctors, or chiropractors who file false or exaggerated claims is acceptable. In the same survey, 1 in 12 adults stated that it is acceptable for someone injured at home to claim a work-related injury for the purpose of collecting workers' compensation benefits.[14]

Often, the nature of the illness or injury claim is an issue. Problems related to stress, myocardial infarction, low back pain, and other health concerns may occur in the work setting. Yet these types of conditions often have etiologic components unrelated to work. Additional exploration of the facts is called for to determine whether the illness will be considered work-related and the worker therefore eligible for compensation benefits.

A host of additional problems emerge when the injured worker has comorbidities. Whereas injury or illness that is work-related is covered by the workers' compensation insurance, any other existing health problems will not be covered. At times, an injured worker may only be able to access care for the illness or injury that is work-related if there is no source of funding to pay for care to treat other health problems. This may lead to diminished health outcomes, a more lengthy period required for recovery and return to work, and, under the best circumstances, fragmented care. Consider, for example, the case of a 20 year old who fell at work and sustained a torn meniscus of the left knee. The workers' compensation insurance paid all costs for diagnosis, arthroscopic surgery, and rehabilitation (in this case physical therapy) following the injury. Unfortunately, this same person fell at home 2 weeks after the initial injury and sustained a similar injury to the right knee. This person had no group health insurance and exceeded the income level to qualify for Medicaid. The client was unable to secure any source of treatment for the second injury because there was no way to pay for care. In the end, the client achieved excellent outcomes in terms of strength and mobility of the left knee but was left with a permanent limitation on the right due to lack of treatment.

In the case of the client just described, even if group health insurance coverage had been available, the client might still have encountered difficulties. Although GHI would cover the expenses for diagnosis and treatment of the knee injury that occurred at home, in all likelihood, the providers of care would be different from the providers managing the care being paid for by workers' compensation. Thus there is potential for considerable fragmentation because two separate systems of care (and of reimbursement for care) are in use. Currently, pilot programs are being developed in four states for which the goal is to develop a model of "24-hour care." The plan is to develop an integrated or "seamless" system of care in which there will be (1) a single bill-paying system, (2) a single doctor, and (3) case management collaboration.[15]

Cost of Workers' Compensation

The premiums required to purchase workers' compensation insurance represent a substantial cost to a business. Since employees do not pay for the insurance, the premium costs, which have been escalating rapidly, must be added in to increase the price for the product or service being produced. Premium costs reflect the increased actual expenses paid out by insurance carriers. For example, from 1990 to 1991, the national average cost of medical benefits per worker increased by almost 12 percent, resulting in an expense of almost $15 million or $150 per worker.[16]

Even the industry created to provide insurance as well as monitor claims has become big business in its own right. Administrative costs add to the problem of premium inflation. Workers' compensation medical charges generally are about twice the cost of comparable charges incurred for off-work injuries. This difference has resulted from lack of cost controls in most workers' compensation programs.[17]

Legislators are focusing on mechanisms to slow the growth of escalating premiums without compromising the quality of care provided. Their efforts tend to focus on ways of strengthening industry safety programs, emphasizing labor-management cooperation, and developing models of health care delivery that will contain costs.

The Case Manager's Role and Workers' Compensation Insurance

The primary goal of the case manager in working with the person who has experienced work-related illness or injury is to facilitate the individual's return to work as rapidly as possible. All the case management strategies discussed throughout this book are applicable. However, in compensation cases, the nature of the client-nurse relationship is different. In essence, the nurse has two clients—the affected worker and the *employer* of the affected worker. Both the employer and nurse share the goal of getting the worker back to work. However, many injured workers may have a low level of motivation to return to work, and malingering as well as outright fraud must be detected. Primary techniques that the nurse case manager uses include:

- Establishing an effective working relationship with the worker in which there is compassion, empathy, and trust.
- Sharing information with the employer to better understand the personality of the worker and discover psychological strategies that might motivate prompt return to work. For example, just a phone call from the employer to the worker made on a regular basis to say hello and provide support and encouragement often has a favorable effect on the worker's attitude about returning to work.

- Exploring how the affected worker's job might be changed to a "light duty" position. If there has been extensive injury or illness, the worker can often return to work sooner if a modified type of work assignment can be created. The case manager must be familiar with the Americans with Disabilities Act (ADA), which creates obligations for employers who have disabled workers returning to work.
- Monitoring the treatment process for appropriateness of interventions and being sensitive to the possibility of excess or "overtreating" by providers.
- Initiating life care planning as needed (this process is discussed in detail in Chapter 9).

The ideal outcome in case management of the injured worker is a recovered and/or rehabilitated employee who returns to work within an appropriate length of time and is able to resume usual activities. Cost-effective services utilized in an efficient manner ensure better treatment standards and continuity of care. The worker is more satisfied. The employer as client is also satisfied and will experience reduced financial burden of escalating insurance premiums.

MOTOR VEHICLE INSURANCE

Most states require that individuals who own motor vehicles assume financial responsibility for any accidents or property damage they cause. The financial responsibility is usually met through the purchase of automobile liability insurance with state-mandated minimum coverage for bodily injury and property damage. Bodily injury coverage provides compensation to another person who is hurt or dies as a result of an automobile accident. The smallest amount of coverage is required by Louisiana, Mississippi, and Oklahoma ($10,000 coverage for one individual injured) and the highest is required by Alaska ($50,000 coverage for one individual injured).[18] Although financial responsibility is ensured by mandatory insurance, the minimums required are far below the $100,000 recommended for bodily injury protection by most experts in the field.

In some states, there is an option to choose who will pay for medical expenses that result from an auto accident. Under the personal injury protection system (PIP), the individual can choose as payer either the auto insurance company or the health insurance company who currently insures the person. Although this may result in substantial cost savings in the price of the automobile policy, it does create a more complex situation in managing the payment for accident-related health care expenses. The individual must verify that the current health insurance policy will pay for auto accident treatment expenses. Any deductibles, copayments, and coverage limits or exclusions of the health insurance policy will still be in effect. If Medicare or Medicaid is the source of health insurance coverage, the PIP option may *not* be selected, as neither government plan allows for it.

According to the National Safety Council, a motor vehicle injury occurs every 16 seconds.[19] It is estimated by the Insurance Information Institute that in 1993 there were 32.8 million motor vehicle accidents with a total cost of $104 billion.[20] Perhaps even more startling is the fact that approximately 373,000 people are hospitalized each year for traumatic brain injury (TBI) most commonly caused by either a motor vehicle accident or violence.[21] Many of these accidents involve relatively young drivers and passengers who are left permanently disabled as a result of the accident.

The case manager working with the client injured in a motor vehicle accident confronts numerous challenges. Many clients face a long period of rehabilitation and may require extensive physical, occupational, speech, cognitive, and psychological therapies. Depending on the type and severity of residual damage, there may be a need for adaptive equipment ranging from wheelchairs, communication devices, and special automobiles or vans to a complete home modification to accommodate the disabled individual. Vocational counseling is a must, since many newly disabled people confront issues of being unable to return to former work and the need to acquire marketable job skills.

Often the case manager is working with a person who is emotionally labile, angry, and cognitively impaired from the accident. Extensive adjustment by the client and family become a priority. Because of the multiplicity of care providers, variety of settings in which treatment occurs, and extended period of time recovery requires, the case manager can expect to have a long-term relationship with the client system.

The most important role of the case manager in these situations is the coordination of the plan of care and services. The case manager (usually employed by the payer of services—the health insurance or automobile insurance carrier) may be the only professional who has a continuing relationship with the individual as he or she progresses through the continuum of care (often acute care to a rehabilitation facility to subacute care or outpatient service if the person returns home). The case manager, as client advocate, will base decisions on the long-term treatment goals. The case manager will continually monitor progress toward goals, negotiate with providers to secure the most cost-effective services available, and may even have to negotiate with the case manager's own employer to persuade them that treatment costs and adaptive equipment or home modifications will lead to better outcomes over time (although they often are more expensive initially).

Policy limits may restrict the range of options available to the client. The case manager needs to be knowledgeable regarding programs and services available in the community, as these can often replace more costly, privately purchased services.

An additional area of concern for case managers working with clients injured in motor vehicle accidents relates to litigation. Often these clients are involved in law suits which, in turn, may involve the testimony or written records of the case manager. For this reason records must be scrupulously accurate, unbiased, and completed in a timely fashion. Confidentiality of records can be maintained by releasing only pertinent information to providers who are authorized to access the information.

Chapter Highlights

* The escalation of health care costs at a pace faster than any other segment of the economy has led to a multitude of managed care strategies to create cost effectiveness without compromising the outcomes of care.
* There are multiple mechanisms to pay for health care. Both public and private sectors are involved. In the public sector, Medicare and Medicaid are currently being revised. In the private sector, the source for paying health care expenses will relate to whether the health care need has arisen from personal factors (group health insurance), is work-related (workers' compensation), or is automobile-related (automobile insurance or GHI).
* The case manager must be thoroughly familiar with the mechanisms for financing health care and the specifics of coverage for any individual's care.
* The case manager is in a unique position to work with the client, the members of the provider team, and the insurer to facilitate delivery of the appropriate type of service in the most economic way. As a result, resources available to the client can be applied to achieve maximum benefit.

References

1. Health Insurance Association of America. (1995). *Source book of health insurance data.* Washington, DC. p. 2.
2. Feldtsein, J. (1993). *Health care economics.* (4th ed.). West Albany, NY: Delmar Publishers. p. 72.
3. Health Insurance Association of America. (1995). *Managed care: Integrating the delivery and financing of health care. Part A.* Washington, DC. p. 40.
4. Ibid., p. 43.

5. Mooney, P., & Lerro, D. (1995/Jan.). Case management using a point of service plan. *Inside Case Management.* 1(10), 6.

6. Clark, M. (1992). *Nursing in the community.* Norwalk, CT: Appleton & Lange. p. 251.

7. Russell-Babbin, K. (speaker). (1994). "Case management: An overview." Villanova, PA: Villanova University.

8. Health Insurance Association of America. *Source book of health insurance data: 1995.* Washington, DC. p. 21.

9. US Health Care Financing Administration. (1994). *The Medicare 1994 handbook.* Washington, DC: US Government Printing Office. p. 39.

10. Clark, M. (1996). *Nursing in the community.* (2d ed.). Stamford, CT: Appleton & Lange. p. 245.

11. US Health Care Financing Administration. (1994/Fall). *Health care financing review.* [on-line].

12. Tyson, L. (1993/Oct. 6). *The costs of failing to reform health care.* Washington, DC: Council of Economic Advisors, The White House. p. 3. [on-line].

13. Office of Disease Prevention and Health Promotion. (1995). *Healthy people 2000.* Health ResponseAbility Systems, Inc. [on-line].

14. Insurance Research Council. (1992/June). Roper Organization Survey. [on-line].

15. Major, M. (1994/Apr, May, June). 24-hour coverage: a concept whose time has come? *The Case Manager.* pp. 62–68.

16. Health Insurance Association of America. (1995). *Managed care: integrating the delivery and financing of health care.* p. 107.

17. Baker, L., & Krueger, A. (1993, Suppl). Twenty-four-hour coverage and workers' compensation insurance. *Health Insurance.* pp. 271–281.

18. Insurance Information Institute. (1995). *The fact book 1996: property/casualty insurance* facts. New York. pp. 115–116.

19. Ibid., p. 84.

20. Ibid., p. 84.

21. Johnson, C. (1995/Nov.). After a brain injury: Clearing up the confusion. *Nursing 95.* 25(11), 39–45.

Skills of the Nurse 4
Case Manager

Nurse case managers must possess a broad range of personal, interpersonal, and management skills in order to carry out their duties. They are now actively involved in almost every type of health care delivery system, including acute care or rehabilitation and subacute facilities as well as home care. Their jobs can be found in traditional indemnity insurance companies as well as managed care organizations. Some case managers work in private practice and may be independent contractors who represent insurance carriers.

Employers seeking case managers often look for experienced critical care or trauma nurses who have been taught to perform rapid head-to-toe assessment. Observant, quick thinking, and quick acting, they can prioritize rapidly and decisively, making use of a sophisticated knowledge base in a particular clinical area. They also delegate effectively, using organizational skills, assertiveness, and diplomacy. These basic skills can be very useful to the nurse assuming the role of case manager.

Sometimes the setting will dictate the knowledge base and clinical expertise required by a candidate. For example, the nurse case manager wishing to work in a rehabilitation center should have a sophisticated knowledge of neurology while a mental health facility will require broad psychiatric knowledge.

This chapter outlines the general skills that the nurse case manager must acquire, fine-tune, and maintain. For the sake of organization we have classified these skills into four categories, although the elements overlap at times. It is important to realize that the skills are not listed in order of importance and in fact many times depend on each other. Figure 4-1 summarizes this information.

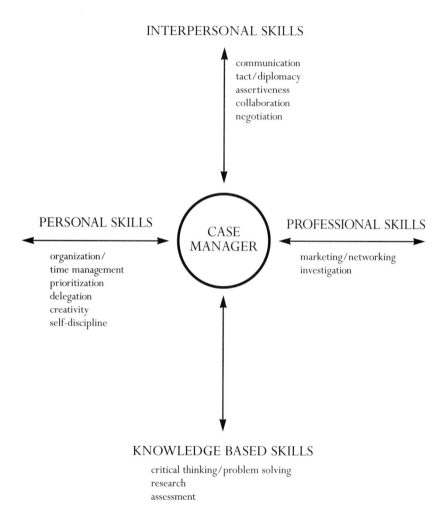

Figure 4-1. *Skills of the nurse case manager*

Upon completion of this chapter you will be able to answer the following questions:

1. What skills need to be developed or acquired to support the role of the nurse case manager?
2. What characteristics of each skill contribute most importantly to effective role development?
3. Which skills are unique to the role of the case manager and which skills apply to many nursing roles?

INTERPERSONAL SKILLS

Communication

Verbal and written communication is an integral part of the case management process. As the person at the center of the multidisciplinary health care team, the case manager must have the ability to interpret extensive and detailed information and disseminate the information to many individuals possessing varied levels of knowledge and understanding. To successfully complete this part of the process, the nurse case manager must develop excellent communication skills to be able to interact with the patient, family members and/or significant others, physicians, other providers of health care services, attorneys, and insurance personnel. The case manager must have the ability to gather information from various sources and, in a succinct and intelligible manner, channel that data to the appropriate people.

Verbal communication

For successful communication to occur, the case manager should have a basic understanding of the communication process. Essentially, this involves listening, observing, processing, and conveying. The case manager must be able to use periods of silence to be able to "read between the lines." Hearing what is not said is as important as listening to the words that are spoken. The case manager should be observant. Accurate interpretation of body language can often fill in the missing pieces of a puzzle. The vast amount of information collected during interviews, record reviews, and observation is then processed and conveyed to the appropriate people so that coordinated, time-effective, and cost-effective treatment can be accomplished across all boundaries.

The case manager must often establish rapport within a very short time span and under very difficult circumstances. In many instances the client has recently been critically injured or diagnosed with a catastrophic illness. The anxiety levels of the client and the family members fearing the unknown are high, so the "stranger"—the case manager—may be viewed as an adversary who will deny requested services or procedures or who will discontinue or decrease benefits. Clients often confuse the role of a nurse case manager with that of an insurance agent who may be perceived, rightly or wrongly, as someone who will save the "company" money at the expense of the client. The nurse case manager's ability to explain her or his role as advocate and to establish trust depends upon communication skills.

Clear definition of terms, use of simple language, and emphasis on the collaborative and advocacy aspects is paramount in establishing rapport. Case managers should also remember that as they observe clients' body language, the clients are observing the case managers.' Without projecting an aura of trust, the information that the case manager obtains during the initial interview may be inaccurate, contradictory, and/or incomplete.

Once good rapport is established, the nurse case manager begins the initial assessment. Providing privacy is extremely important to reinforce trust and establish an area conducive to a free flow of communication. If the interview is not in the client's home, you should attempt to provide as much privacy as possible by closing the curtain (if the client is hospitalized), speaking softly, and letting the client know that you respect his or her privacy and that, if necessary, you will discuss certain aspects of his or her status at another time.

A comprehensive assessment requires excellent interviewing skills. A good interview involves obtaining the maximum amount of information with a minimum amount of questioning. Clients who feel they are getting "the third degree" may become hostile, threatened, and less than forthcoming. Asking open-ended questions will encourage the client to elaborate. Open-ended questions allow the client freedom to respond with more detail and to express attitude and behavior, whereas closed-ended questions result in a *yes* or *no* response. A closed-ended question would be, "Do you like your job?" An open-ended question such as "How do you feel about returning to work?" would elicit a more detailed response regarding the client's motivation to return to work, the relationship with the employer, and possibly the client's thoughts about career goals. The experienced interviewer will use a combination of open- and closed-ended questions. Too many open-ended questions may lead the conversation away from the main subject and result in a discussion of irrelevant topics. The case manager's communication skills must keep the interview on course and within the time frames allowed.

Cultural influences on communication

The nurse case manager should have a basic knowledge of cultural differences and a thorough knowledge of the culture of the specific client population. Certain questions are inappropriate or may cause embarrassment in various cultures. Behavior patterns and/or family involvement vary among cultures and may lead case managers to draw incorrect conclusions if they do not understand the culture of their clients. Ethnocentrism (the belief that one's own culture is superior) or cultural blindness (ignoring cultural differences) may result in a distortion of communication, undermine the nurse/client relationship, and result in a plan of care that will fail to produce the desired outcomes.[1]

The case manager should be aware that culture affects health both directly and indirectly. Direct effects involve specific practices related to diet or practices prescribed to restore health or prevent illness. Indirect effects involve the cultural definition of health and illness. For example, certain behavior patterns that may be perceived as signs of mental illness in one culture may be viewed as normal in another culture. Some cultures view a diagnosis of mental illness as shameful, something to hide. The nurse case manager coordinating care for the client with mental illness should be aware that expression of feelings and confrontation, which are encouraged in Western psychotherapy, are prohibited behaviors in certain cultures; encouragement of these behaviors therefore will be an ineffective mode of treatment.[2]

Cultural differences are also found within the context in which a message is conveyed. Certain cultures, such as that considered American, are *low context*. A message is relayed in the words that are used. In a *high context* culture, such as in Japan, the message is conveyed by the context of the situation rather than the words used. For example, if the nurse case manager asks a client when she or he is planning to schedule a follow-up appointment with the physician, certain cultures would dictate that the response given would be the one expected by the case manager. Thus, the client may tell the case manager that he or she will call tomorrow. When the case manager contacts the client a week later and finds that the appointment is still not scheduled, the case manager may view the client as non-compliant and unmotivated. In reality, the client's response was within the context of her or his culture, where "tomorrow" can mean "some time in the near future."[3]

As with words, gestures can convey different meanings in different cultures. For example, "clients from India would be highly insulted if the soles of one's shoes were directed towards them." In Indian culture the soles of the shoes are considered dirty, and directing the sole of a shoe toward the person, would be analogous to "spitting in someone's face in the United States."[4]

Knowledge of cultural practices may also enhance the case manager's ability to assess motivation and/or malingering. As an example, there was a client who injured his back in a work-related accident. The employer, the insurance carrier, and the physician suspected malingering but were unable to prove it. During the initial interview, the client stated that he was Muslim and prayed several times per day. Through knowledge of the way in which the Muslims pray, and with further discussion with the client, it was evident that this client was able to kneel on the floor and flex his back without any apparent problems. After mentioning this to the physician, who concurred that the client's complaints of pain were questionable, treatment was discontinued and the client was released to return to work.

Since all communication involves interpretation within the context of our own individual perceptions, misunderstanding and ambiguity often accompany verbal conversation between two people. Paraphrasing, summarizing, and clarifying what the client has stated ensures that the case manager is processing the information correctly and minimizes any ambiguity that might otherwise result. In addition, by summarizing, the case manager demonstrates that he or she has been listening to the client and is interested in what the client has to say. A pitfall to avoid is interjecting judgment within the confines of the response. For example, a client states, "My employer keeps calling to ask when I'm returning to work. He thinks that I'm making this up." The nurse case manager might respond with, "You sound angry" or "Your employer is only interested in your well-being." Those responses may sound judgmental or leading and may cause the client to become defensive. A more appropriate response would be, "Can you describe how you feel when your employer calls?"

Communication is an art as well as a skill. The ability to send and receive messages, gather information and disseminate the data, without confusing the intent or misinforming the receiver, is the solid foundation on which the case management process is built.

Written communication

Much of the case management process requires written communication. The case manager must be able to compile all the data received during the initial interview and summarize it in a comprehensive, succinct report. The initial report follows the format of the initial assessment tool (see Appendix I for examples of reports). Progress reports, which are usually required every 30 days, generally describe the activity during that period, the client's current status and the case manager's recommendations.

The case manager must have an excellent command of the English language and the ability to summarize large amounts of information without distortion or judgment. The written report is forwarded to the referral source, who in many instances is a nonmedical person unfamiliar with medical terminology. The report should use nontechnical terminology and should contain clear, concise, factual, and accurate documentation.

In essence, the written report is an anecdotal record which documents, summarizes, analyzes, and synthesizes the verbal and nonverbal data. The report includes recommendations and projected time frames based on input from all members of the health care team. The payer refers to the report when deciding appropriateness of care, and the report can be subpoenaed for any legal purposes including litigation.

The nurse case manager's written communication skills are also required for letter writing. As the person negotiating costs with various providers, the case manager is responsible for documenting the negotiated rates. The nature of the item or service requested must be clearly defined, with the approved time frames and negotiated costs.

As an example, a nurse case manager receives authorization to coordinate skilled nursing care for a client for 8 hours per day, 7 days per week. The exact time frames may be indefinite, and the referral source indicates that approval would be given for 2 weeks and then reevaluated. The case manager contacts a nursing agency and requests LPN-level nursing at a negotiated rate of $33 per hour. A letter of documentation is then sent to the nursing agency to confirm all aspects of the case. The case manager with poor writing skills may send a letter stating, "LPN visits at $33 per hour, 8 hours per day for 2 weeks." The case manager with excellent writing skills will generate a letter stating, "LPN visits, 8 hours per day, 7 days per week. Start date is 12/1/XX. End date is 12/29/XX. The negotiated rate is $33 per hour, including weekends and holidays. Continued coverage will be reevaluated during the week of 12/25/XX. If coverage continues to be approved, these rates will remain in effect." The second letter does not allow for misinterpretation, as it clearly documents what is authorized and for how long.

Tact and Diplomacy

Tact and diplomacy, necessary components of the case manager's arsenal, are used here interchangeably to mean the ability to handle a delicate situation appropriately. The nurse case manager needs to develop tact when communicating with the various members of the multidisciplinary health care team, when communicating with attorneys, when delegating tasks, when seeking information from the client or family members, and when requesting authorization from insurance carriers. Coming across as judgmental, authoritative, controlling, and superior will alienate everyone and make objectives difficult, if not impossible, to accomplish. The nurse case manager, at the center of the multidisciplinary team, is responsible for maintaining a smooth flow of communication, continuity of care, and positive outcomes.

With today's rapidly shifting health care environment, physicians often feel they are increasingly losing control. Their ability to design treatment plans is limited by the tight reins the insurance industry is placing on their decision-making power. Managed care organizations are prohibiting physicians from divulging all treatment options to their patients, information which may lead to an increase in the cost of care.[5] Critical pathways and MAPs are outlining treatment protocols that many physicians are calling "cook book medicine." Because of this perception of a changing medical atmosphere, physicians may take offense if the nurse case manager appears to be dictating the physician's treatment plan. An adversarial relationship can easily emerge, which results in poor communication or collaborative efforts to the detriment of the client.

The art of diplomacy will aid the case manager in developing positive communication, a collaborative relationship, and respect for the case manager's input. During the initial contact with the physician, the nurse case manager should state his or her role, inform the physician represented, and clearly communicate the goal of establishing a collaborative relationship to produce positive outcomes for the physician and the client. Through a tactful approach, a positive relationship will increase the case manager's ability to obtain necessary information and treatment recommendations. In addition, the physician will be more apt to respect the case manager's input and suggestions for an alternative treatment plan.

As an example, I had a client who was discharged home on IV antibiotics, to be infused via heparin lock every 6 hours. The client's significant other was unable to learn the infusion technique, which meant coordinating six skilled nursing visits per day. I spoke with the physician about inserting a central line and ordering a CADD pump, which has a computer chip that needs to be reset once daily. The pump automatically infuses the antibiotic at the set time. This would reduce the skilled nursing visits from six to one daily. Since the client also had poor veins, it was likely that he would need to have the heparin lock changed frequently. With a central line, no line change would be required. Since a positive relationship with this physician had already been established, he listened to my recommendations and agreed that inserting the central line would be both cost-effective and better for the patient. Had an adversarial relationship existed, the physician might have been defensive, thinking that I was trying to tell him how to treat. The outcome would have been more costly and might have been more uncomfortable for the client.

Tact and diplomacy are also necessary when speaking with attorneys. When a nurse case manager receives a workers' compensation claim, attorney approval must be received prior to contacting the client. Many attorneys view the nurse case manager as the person who is going to deny treatment, decrease benefits, and encourage the client's physician to release the client to return to work. Again, a positive relationship can be established through clearly stating the goal of a collaborative relationship. The nurse case manager who can convince the attorney that his or her role is to assist the client in receiving the best possible treatment and not to force clients to return to work before they are physically able is the one who will be successful in receiving approval to proceed.

Diplomacy is one of the main ingredients necessary to accomplish set goals. The nurse case manager who needs to delegate work in the course of coordinating care will complete this task successfully if she or he communicates the needs clearly, succinctly, and tactfully. The receiver will accept the challenges and/or increased work load with a positive attitude when the request is perceived as part of a collaborative effort, not an order.

The nurse case manager deals with a myriad of personality styles while coordinating an effective plan of care. Within the circle of providers nurse case managers will encounter those who thrive on real or imagined positions of power. Flexibility, along with diplomacy and tact, will often bring the desired results. The case manager who can establish rapport and develop insight into the other person's personality traits will be a sensitive communicator.

For example, claims adjusters can think that their authority is being usurped when case managers recommend care that is not exactly in accordance with the insurance plan. The case manager who can approach this situation armed with confidence, an appropriate rationale, cost savings data, and communication finesse will avoid conflict and allow the claims adjuster to listen openly.

Assertiveness Skills

Within any personal or working relationship, conflict is bound to occur. People deal with friction in several ways, including assertiveness, aggressiveness, passive aggression, or passivity. Assertiveness and aggressiveness are not synonymous. *Assertiveness* is defined as "setting goals, acting on these goals in a clear and consistent manner, and taking responsibility for the consequences of those actions."[6] Assertive behavior involves honesty and eye contact and avoids infringing on the rights of others. Assertive behavior demands control over outbursts of anger, temper tantrums, crying, or other behavior patterns that exhibit lack of professionalism. *Aggressive behavior*, however, seeks to "dominate, humiliate, deprecate, or embarrass others for the purpose of exerting power."[7] The person exhibiting aggressive behavior is usually insensitive to others' feelings and uses sarcasm and accusatory statements to maintain a position of power. *Passive aggressive behavior* is the quiet use of aggression. The passive aggressive person is usually manipulative and controlling. A case manager using passive aggressive behavior would intentionally delay returning a phone call to a person considered an authority figure. *Passive behavior* is exhibited by the person who wants to avoid confrontation at any cost. The passive person cannot express opinions and becomes anxious, withdrawn, and nonverbal during conflict.

The most effective way to resolve conflict is through assertive behavior. The nurse case manager who uses assertiveness in conjunction with tact will resolve conflict in a timely fashion and will avoid succumbing to aggressive behavior. Assertiveness brings with it open dialogue and exchange of information, avoids defensiveness, and encourages compromise. People who exhibit assertive behavior patterns are respected and admired as professionals; their recommendations are seriously considered, and their resolutions for conflict are listened to.

Most assertive statements begin with *I*. "*I* statements" imply that the speaker is taking responsibility for her or his feelings and position in the conflict. Examples such as, "I feel, I believe, I expect" are clear and direct expressions of feelings, opinions, or desires. Statements that begin with *You*, such as, "You think, You feel, You are" may place the listener on the defensive. *You* statements make a judgment and are assumptive, since nobody can be exactly sure of what another person is thinking or of what another's behavior is implying. Although most assertive behavior patterns involve statements, questions are often necessary. Questions that begin with *How* are neutral, are perceived as collaborative, and will elicit information. *Why* questions seek explanations or assessments and will often place the other person on the defensive.[8]

As with all dialogue, verbal and nonverbal communication must match. Tone of voice, posture, and facial expression should be congruent with the verbal message. If the nonverbal behavior conflicts with the spoken words, mixed messages are sent. This results in confusion and/or misinterpretation on the part of the listener.

Assertiveness also involves the use of silence. The assertive person will respect the other person's input and listen to what is being said. Interrupting, commenting, showing annoyance, or correcting may elicit defensiveness, close off communication, and prolong the conflict. To maintain an open dialogue, it may be necessary to respond to an angry outburst at a later time, when the listener may be more receptive.

Collaboration

The nurse case manager is responsible for resolving conflict, encouraging and maintaining open communication, facilitating a positive flow of ideas, and achieving high-quality, cost-effective outcomes for everyone involved in the client's care. To accomplish these goals, the nurse case manager must possess collaborative skills in addition to assertiveness, tact, and communication skills.

As a result of the paradigm shifts in health care today, the delivery system has evolved into one of collaborative care. *Collaboration* is described as two or more people working together toward a common goal. Input is equal, and responsibility is shared. Shared knowledge and ideas broaden the scope of information and result in a comprehensive plan of care.[9] No longer is the physician making all treatment decisions. In today's health care arena, treatment plans are a result of equal input from all providers of care.

The nurse case manager is at the center of the collaborative circle and must possess the skills to encourage open dialogue and input from all members of the team to ensure that the focus of the collaborative effort remains working together. If the focus switches to a power struggle among the members, conflict will arise, communication will shut down, and the efforts to design a comprehensive care plan will fail.

For female nurse case managers, interacting and collaborating with authority figures, most of whom are still male, can be difficult. Historically, females in general, and nurses specifically, have been rewarded for obedience, courtesy, and performance of tasks. Although the women's movement has opened many opportunities for females, independent thinking and positions of authority are typically regarded as male perks. Since nursing continues to be primarily a female profession, society in general does not assign nurses to roles with power, autonomy, or leadership. The socialization pattern of physicians and nurses has been one of dominant/submissive behavior. Economic and educational differences between physicians and nurses perpetuate this pattern.[10] Add to this the physician's perception of losing control, due to constraints placed on decision making from managed care organizations, and it is no wonder that the current medical environment is not conducive to collaborative efforts and shared decision making.

Despite the compounded issues which make the nurse case manager's role as collaborator more difficult, with the appropriate demeanor, skills, and professionalism, successful outcomes can be and are achieved. To become proficient in the process of collaboration, the nurse case manager must first perfect skills of communication and assertiveness. Successful outcomes of collaborative care depend upon the ability to interact with others in a positive and productive manner.

When the physician and others in positions of authority see how the case management process can bring about positive outcomes, the case manager's credibility is increased. It is through successful case management that delays in treatment and fragmentation of care are avoided. The client receives the highest quality of care which is cost-effective and timely. As the physician or other professional develops trust and respect for the nurse case manager and realizes that a collaborative effort will enhance everyone's ability to care for the patient, a positive working relationship will replace the power struggle that might otherwise exist.

Negotiation

Negotiation is simply the act of arriving at a compromise pertaining to a situation involving two or more people. Each side of the negotiation strives to persuade the other that its view is the better one. The successful negotiator has charisma, good interpersonal relationships, flexibility, and negotiating skills. These qualities are not inborn but can be learned and become perfected through practice and experience. An inherent aspect of successful negotiation is a strong foundation of trust between or among the parties involved, similarity of goals, and knowledge of what is being negotiated.[11] Prior to developing skills in negotiation, the nurse case manager must perfect the skills of interpersonal relationships and research.

The nurse case manager, as coordinator and facilitator, often must negotiate on behalf of the client, the insurance carrier, the physician, or other providers of health care. Much of the coordination process involves negotiating costs with various providers. To effect significant cost savings without compromising quality, the nurse case manager must develop excellent negotiating skills. Negotiation is also necessary for the role of client advocate. If the nurse case manager brings a plan of care to the carrier that is not entirely within the scope of the benefit policy, approval of the plan as extracontractual will depend on the case manager's ability to negotiate or persuade the claims adjuster that it would be more profitable to authorize rather than deny the treatment. When the nurse case manager has a client injured at work, negotiation skills will be paramount in discussing and recommending modified or light-duty jobs.

Negotiation involves four steps which will be explored briefly in this section. (See Chapter 7 for an in-depth discussion of the negotiation process.) The first step in the negotiating process is researching the answers to "The Three Knows" and begins before the initial contact is made. It is difficult, if not impossible, to convince somebody about an issue when your knowledge is limited.

- *Know what it is.* To negotiate successfully the nurse case manager must have a clear understanding of what is being negotiated.
- *Know who it is.* Without a comprehensive and an accurate knowledge base regarding the client, the provider, the payer, and the policy benefits, successful negotiation will be difficult or impossible.
- *Know what it costs.* The nurse case manager must research the average cost of the various services, equipment, and supplies in the area in which she or he is coordinating care. Without this information negotiation will be futile.

The second step in the negotiation process involves contacting the payer. The nurse case manager discusses his or her recommendations with the claims adjuster. Nurse case managers cannot proceed with coordinating care until they receive approval.

Once approval from the payer is received, the nurse case manager proceeds with the third step in the negotiating process, which is contacting the provider. Establishing good rapport, remaining flexible, and realizing that compromise is inherent in the negotiation process will produce successful outcomes.

The fourth step in the negotiation process is documentation of what has been negotiated. If the negotiation process involves coordinating services, equipment, or supplies at a reduced rate, the nurse case manager must document the negotiated rate clearly, succinctly, and accurately. Refer to the previous discussion of communication skills and letter writing to review the method of documenting and the implications of incomplete documentation.

PROFESSIONAL SKILLS

Marketing and Networking

Independent case managers sell case management services to insurance carriers, third-party administrators, and large, self-insured corporations. Within the confines of case management, the term *marketing* is usually used instead of the term *selling* as a means of maintaining an air of professionalism. *Networking*, which is the process of developing and maintaining professional contacts and relationships, is an ongoing and necessary process in nursing case management in general and is particularly important in the external nurse case management arena. Because marketing and networking are practiced primarily within external case management, a brief overview here is followed by a more in-depth discussion in Chapter 7.

Many people feel that people are either born with an ability to sell or are not. Many believe that a person cannot learn the necessary skills involved in becoming a successful marketer. Although it is true that some people seem naturally able to persuade others through charisma and/or inborn personality traits, the ability to sell successfully a product or a service can be and is a learned technique. The nurse case manager who takes on the role of marketer will succeed with fine-tuned skills of communication, tact, assertiveness, research, and negotiation.

Of prime importance is an in-depth knowledge of the service or product that you are marketing. The nurse working as a marketer for a subacute facility will find it difficult to persuade case managers and insurance carriers to use that specific subacute facility if he or she is unable to explain the benefits of subacute in general, the specific population best served, and why that facility is better than the others. Even the person who can "sell air conditioners in the North Pole" won't succeed without knowing what an air conditioner is or who lives in the North Pole.

Networking is an essential part of marketing and case management in general. The marketer with a comprehensive knowledge base and excellent skills in interpersonal relationships needs an audience to market to. The nurse case manager working within an acute-care facility needs to establish relationships with ancillary staff members. An integral part of successful outcomes from collaborative care planning is the positive relationships formed within the multidisciplinary team.

Investigation

A very harsh reality in health care today is the growing number of fraudulent cases. "Estimates from the General Accounting Office, the National Association of Insurance Commissioners, as well as other industry groups, state that all types of insurance fraud cost U.S. insurers upward of $100 billion every year. Roughly 10 percent of all claims nationwide involve some type of fraud. Direct costs attributable to insurance claims fraud alone amount to nearly $850 per U.S. family."[12]

The nurse case manager, especially when working with clients injured in work-related accidents or motor vehicle accidents, is often the first line of defense against fraud. Although the notion of "tender loving care" and patient advocacy is inherent in nursing, the fact is that clients can be malingerers, and some will file fraudulent claims to try to "milk" the system. As the person representing the insurance carrier or employer, with the objectives of coordinating appropriate and timely medical care and assisting the client to return to work, assessing for possible fraud remains an integral part of the nurse case manager's role.

Most claims are legitimate. However, although the total percentage of fraudulent claims is small, that percentage translates into a large amount of misused time and money. Unfortunately, many employers, insurance claims adjusters, and nurse case managers have become cynical. As the problem with fraud increases, it has become more acceptable to believe that the majority of claims are not legitimate. The experienced nurse case manager must maintain an objective viewpoint regarding the caseload and the people involved.

The nurse case manager should remember to be a nurse, not a detective. Various guidelines should be adhered to when suspecting fraud, as needed. These guidelines include attention to detail, clarification of information, appropriate recommendations, and accurate documentation. The case manager who reports possible fraud too frequently will lose credibility. The case manager who never suspects fraud may be perceived as ineffectual and gullible. Since investigational skills are used primarily by the external case manager, this area will be explored in depth in Chapter 7.

KNOWLEDGE-BASED SKILLS

Although knowledge is not a skill per se, acquiring the appropriate knowledge and knowing where to find information are. In the past, a person was considered an "expert" who knew everything about one specific subject. The expert today knows where to find the answers. Because of the information explosion, it is impossible for one person to have all the answers. The nurse case manager, as a referral source, must be equipped with comprehensive resources. (See Appendix II for a list of commonly referred to resources.)

The nurse case manager must also have a thorough understanding of the statutes and regulations as they pertain to the client's insurance. Workers' compensation laws vary from state to state, as does motor vehicle insurance. The nurse case manager who is working with clients injured in work-related accidents or in motor vehicle accidents will be ineffective without the appropriate knowledge base.

The specialist nurse case manager must have sophisticated knowledge in a specific area of nursing. Ironically, as medicine is moving toward the generalist (e.g., family physician as gatekeeper), nursing case management is moving away from the generalist. High-risk pregnancies, neonates, and pediatrics are highly specialized areas. Clients with problems associated with mental health or substance abuse are also referred to the nurse case manager specialist. As the technology increases for treating head injury and spinal cord injury, rehabilitation case management nurses are becoming more specialized. Since HIV/AIDS is evolving from an acute disease into a chronic illness with a multitude of treatment options, this too is rapidly becoming a specialized area.

Critical Thinking and Problem Solving Skills

As nurses in general increase their autonomy, and the role of the case manager expands, the need for critical thinking and problem solving increases proportionately. In the past, nurses generally developed short-term goals, and decision making was an individual process. Long-term potential problems were rarely identified, and problem-solving techniques were used only in crisis intervention.[13]

In today's health care environment, with its emphasis on prevention and critical pathways, the need to identify potential problems becomes an integral part of the process. Positive outcomes depend on the successful resolution of the problems. Since the role of the nurse case manager is to coordinate care and effectuate a smooth and time-effective delivery system across all boundaries, her or his competence depends on skills of problem identification and timely resolution.

Problem solving is not synonymous with decision making. Although the two processes can depend on each other, there are times when problem solving does not require decision making, and decisions do not always involve a problem.[14] Many times problem solving is instinctual or habitual and does not involve a level of conscious mental processing, such as grabbing a stationary object to prevent a fall. Within the scope of case management, an example of a nonproblematic decision would be coordinating the purchase of DME, such as a hospital bed. The decision to purchase the bed has no bearing on a future course of action. However, the decision either to purchase or to rent the bed will require problem solving. The nurse case manager must project the long-term needs of the client. Will the client need the hospital bed for more than a few months? Is the client expected to improve or deteriorate? What is the payer's benefit policy? If the decision to rent rather than purchase is appropriate, will the provider agree to a rental toward purchase? In essence, "decision making is the behavior exhibited in selecting and implementing a course of action from among alternatives that may or may not involve a problem."[15]

The first step in problem solving is identification of the problem. With the advent of critical pathways and MAPs, early identification of problems has been enhanced through the use of variances. The critical pathway describes specific outcomes along a timeline. If the outcome is not completed by the projected time, a variance occurs. Breaking down the problem to its simplest level will allow for an organized, accurate, and timely resolution.

The second step in problem solving is classification of the problem. The ability to categorize appropriately is contingent upon the nurse case manager's prioritizing skills. Problems can be classified as potential, actual, or critical. Potential problems are those that may occur in the future but do not necessarily need immediate attention. Actual problems may need immediate attention. Critical problems require crisis intervention.[16] The nurse case manager who has not perfected prioritizing skills may have excellent problem-solving skills and yet fail to initiate resolution of variances appropriately. If he or she spends time resolving potential problems, the actual problems may become critical. Similarly, the nurse case manager who has superior prioritizing skills and lacks the ability to problem-solve will also fail to achieve the desired outcomes.

There are various methods of problem solving. The least desirable, and most often used by the those with little or no experience, is trial and error. The case manager using this method will try one solution after another until the problem is resolved. This process is not only time consuming and costly but can be detrimental to the client and will make the nurse case manager appear ineffectual.

Another method of problem solving is experimentation. This technique may involve limited trials or pilot projects and, if used appropriately, can lead to major changes in a system or process. Examples of experimentation as a problem-solving technique include the pilot programs designed within many of the acute care facilities first attempting to incorporate case management into their systems. Through encouraging creativity, building on positive outcomes, and eliminating practices that did not result in positive change, this experimentation produced the case management process as a successful means of delivering care in those institutions.

Critiquing is another method of problem solving. As the person at the center of the multidisciplinary team, the nurse case manager often uses this method, which entails listening to input from the other members of the team and offering constructive feedback. This process is frequently used when there is difficulty concerning problem identification. It is the case manager's role to prevent a breakdown in communication and to maintain the group focus.

The metaphor-based technique and brainstorming are two frequently used methods of problem solving within a group structure. The metaphor-based method is highly creative, evokes original ideas through association, and uses fantasy or symbolism in analyzing and resolving a problem. The group discards usual solutions for a problem and designs new resolutions from a completely different viewpoint. For example, an elderly client has frequent readmissions due to repeated falls at home. The multidisciplinary team would imagine themselves as the elderly client. They would fantasize how they might prevent falling. They might imagine themselves floating above the floor or having magical powers to stop a fall in progress. These metaphors might be translated into performing a home assessment to ensure that scatter rugs and the like are not the cause of repeated injury. Possibly the solution is simply providing a walker or a cane to assist with poor balance. The magical power analogy may require referral to community resources for additional home assistance.

Brainstorming, similar to metaphor-based problem solving, requires creativity, new ways of looking at a problem, and encouraging all members to participate. Successful brainstorming requires withholding judgment, exploring any and all suggestions, generating large numbers of ideas, and expanding on other participants' suggestions. At the conclusion of the brainstorming session, the suggestions are evaluated to determine the degree of feasibility and the pros and cons.

The actual process of successful problem solving involves eight steps. These steps are problem identification, information gathering, analysis of the information, developing a solution, considering the consequences, making a decision, implementing the decision, and evaluating the solution.[17] The main ingredients needed to accomplish these tasks successfully include excellent communication and organizational skills, flexibility, and a lack of preconceived ideas.

Research Skills

Fundamental to being a sleuth is acquiring the ability to discover or locate information. Understanding models of data collection and analysis, and interpretation of the findings, are essential elements in instituting change or resolving problems. In its broadest sense, research is finding solutions to problems, which can then be predicted or explained.[18]

Research is also the means of enhancing the body of knowledge to elevate case management into a highly regarded profession. As with nursing in general, the embryonic stages of case management evolution involved the description of the roles and characteristics of the nurse case manager. The next step in establishing nursing case management as a true specialty is to focus on problems in the delivery system. The theories derived from research form standard resolutions to these problems. Research, as one of the main ingredients for enhancing the power of a profession, has been incorporated into the ANA's "Standards of Professional Performance." In 1991 the ANA mandated that professional nurses use research findings in practice.[19] The ANA defines research as "developing knowledge about health and the promotion of health over the full life span, care of persons with health problems and disabilities, and nursing actions to enhance the ability of individuals to respond effectively to actual or potential health problems."[20]

There are two basic categories of research. The first category is basic research, which is gaining knowledge for the sake of knowledge. Applied research, the second category, applies the knowledge gained to everyday situations. Case management research is generally applied research, as it is used to ask and answer questions regarding the care of the client in the health care delivery system. Within these two basic categories are seven types of research. They are as follows:

1. Historical—collection and assessment of data regarding past events
2. Exploratory—initial studies designed to develop or refine a problem
3. Assessing—tests of how well a policy or program is working
4. Descriptive—accurate identification of characteristics of people or events, and the frequency at which they occur.
5. Experimental—tests of relationships between variables through control of an independent variable with random assignment of subjects to different conditions
6. Quasi-experimental—tests of relationships between variables through independent control of a variable, but without random assignment of subjects to different conditions
7. Correlational—exploration of the interrelationships among variables without active intervention.[21]

Nursing case management research can incorporate all seven types. The appropriate type depends on the particulars of the problem.

Regardless of the type of research used, a basic process must be adhered to. As with problem solving, the first step in the research process is defining the problem. Once the problem is identified, the researcher develops an hypothesis, or assumption that can be tested. Using a variety of techniques, data are collected, compiled, analyzed, and interpreted. The final step in the research process is drawing conclusions from the interpreted data collection.[22]

The analyzed data can provide the framework for projecting time-lines for developing critical pathways, evaluating treatment plans, predicting variances and outcomes, and justifying recommendations. The information can also be used to develop new programs, assist in problem-solving techniques, and enhance the overall goal of providing high-quality care in a cost-effective manner, across all boundaries of the health care delivery system.

Assessment

A complete, comprehensive assessment is critical to achieve positive outcomes and facilitate successful case management. The initial client assessment is a time-consuming process that requires data collection from a variety of sources, a broad knowledge base, and excellent communication skills.

Through collaboration with all health care providers, and interaction with the patient and family, the case manager collects data to complete a comprehensive assessment of the medical/nursing/psychosocial/spiritual/environmental/vocational status and needs of the patient. The strategies for data collection include reviewing existing records, interviewing the client and/or family, and observing the client-family situation.

Case management often is not "hands on" nursing. The nurse case manager might have to assess a client's status using only visual and auditory cues. A detailed, thorough, and appropriate initial assessment tool provides a guide to focus on the specifics of the client's status, current problems, and medical history. The assessment tool used will depend upon the source of the referral. For example, the initial assessment of a client who was injured at work will differ from that of a client with a non-work-related injury. The majority of injuries that occur at work are not catastrophic in nature. The assessment will require obtaining detailed information regarding a description of the injury, the immediate and follow-up treatment, and existing comorbidities that might have a direct impact on the client's healing process, such as a diagnosis of diabetes.

If a case manager were doing an initial assessment with a client who had sustained a torn rotator cuff of the right shoulder, collecting detailed information concerning all body systems would, in most instances, be irrelevant and unrelated. Remember that when a case manager is working with a client who was injured at work, the insurance carrier is responsible only for health problems that are directly related to the injury. If the client had a history of recurrent urinary tract infection, the past treatments and current medical recommendations would have no bearing on the client's torn rotator cuff. However, the case manager should identify a preexisting shoulder injury. When a worker exacerbates a preexisting injury, the employer can use a specially designed fund to assist with expenses related to the injury. It would also be important to determine if the client were right-hand dominant. An injury to the right shoulder of a left-hand dominant client might have more positive outcomes than the same injury sustained by a right-hand dominant client.

As important as the medical information is a comprehensive educational and vocational history, including skills assessment, determination of career goals, and a job analysis. Since it is often more costly for the workers' compensation carrier to reimburse lost wages than to pay for the medical treatment, the primary goal is frequently a timely return to work. Detailed information regarding job duties, transferrable skills, availability of light duty work, and motivation to return to work would have an important impact on the goal of a timely return to work. The case manager will need to assess the client's functional limitations and obtain a job description with physical requirements. Questions regarding limitations would examine the client's ability to perform the following: walking, climbing, sitting, squatting, bending, twisting, turning, reaching, lifting, pulling, and pushing; a nurse case manager would also assess visual, auditory and other sensory changes.

To evaluate a client diagnosed with a non-work-related injury or illness, the case manager needs a clear understanding of the particular terms of the client's insurance carrier (indemnity, managed care, self-insured), whether to use a PPO, and any policy limits. The assessment will have a strong medical focus, with minimal information regarding work history. Asking appropriate questions, observing verbal and nonverbal cues, and drawing precise conclusions allow the case manager to make an accurate assessment.

See Tables 4-1 and 4-2 for examples of initial assessment tools for the client injured in a work-related accident and for the client with a medical diagnosis. For the client who sustains a catastrophic injury at work, the inital assessment should contain comprehensive and detailed information regarding both medical and vocational data. The assessment tool for such a client would be a combination of both tables.

Table 4-1. Initial Assessment Tool for a Client with Workers' Compensation Insurance

Name:_____	Referral source:_____
Insured:_____	Address:_____
Policy #:_____	_____
Social Security #:_____	_____
Address:_____	_____
Phone:_____	Phone:_____ Fax:_____
Fax:_____	
	Contact person:_____
Date of birth:_____	Date of injury:_____
Diagnosis:_____	

I. Introduction
1. Reason for referral:_____
2. Place of interview/parties present:_____

Text continues on page 84

3. Attorney:_____   Approval: ☐ yes   ☐ no
   Address:_____

   _____

   Phone:_____   Fax:_____
4. Employer:
   Address:_____

   _____

   Phone:_____   Fax:_____
   Contact person:_____

II. History of Injury
Date of injury:_____
Description of injury:_____

_____

Hospital
   Name:_____
   Address:_____
   Treated in emergency room:
          yes ☐   no ☐ Ambulance: yes ☐   no ☐
   Admitted: yes ☐   no ☐
   Physician_____
      Address:_____

      _____

      _____

      Phone:_____   Fax:_____
   Hospitalization treatment:_____

   _____

   Surgery:_____
   Date:_____
   Discharge date:_____   Discharged to:_____
   Outpatient treatment:_____

III. Current Status
Height:_____ Weight: _____ Loss/gain since injury:_____
Hand dominance:_____
Medications:_____
Physician(s):_____

Date of last appointment:_____ Date of next appointment:_____

Therapists:_____

Frequency:_____

Modalities:_____

Subjective complaints:_____

Objective data:_____

Transportation

    Drive: yes ☐   no ☐   shift ☐   automatic ☐

Equipment/supply needs:_____

Functional limitations:_____

	Limitation	No limitation	Explanation
Walking	☐	☐	_____
Climbing	☐	☐	_____
Sitting	☐	☐	_____
Squatting	☐	☐	_____
Bending	☐	☐	_____
Twisting/turning	☐	☐	_____
Reaching	☐	☐	_____
Lifting	☐	☐	_____
Vision	☐	☐	_____
Hearing	☐	☐	_____
Sensory changes	☐	☐	_____

IV. Medical History

1. Past serious or prolonged illnesses (dates): _____

   _____

2. Past surgeries (dates; hospitalization; physician):_____

   _____

3. Past workers' compensation injuries (dates; length of time out of work; residual symptoms): _____

   _____

4. Past motor vehicle injuries (dates; residual symptoms):_____

   _____

5. Substance use and/or abuse:_____

6. Pertinent family history:_____

7. Chronic illnesses (diabetes, hypertension, etc., include medications):

   _____

V. Psychosocial & Economic Status

1. Marital status:_____   Marital history:_____

   Spouse's occupation:_____

2. Dependents (number, ages, custodial parent):_____

   _____

3. Relationship observed with family members/significant others:

   _____

4. Appearance:_____

5. Attitude observed:_____

6. Pain behavior observed:_____

7. Client's home: own ☐   rent ☐   type_____

   Amount of mortgage or rent:_____

   Barriers:_____

   Status of neighborhood:_____

8. Interests/hobbies:_____

9. Unusual expenses or debt (credit card, automobile, etc.):_____

   _____

VI. Education

1. Highest grade completed:_____

   High school diploma: yes ☐   no ☐

   GED: yes ☐   no ☐

   College degree: yes ☐   no ☐

2. Vocational school: yes ☐   no ☐

   Graduated: yes ☐   no ☐

   Subject:_____

3. Certificates/diplomas/licenses:_____

4. Military service: yes ☐   no ☐

5. Primary language:_____

6. Literate in English: yes ☐   no ☐

   Approximate reading level:_____

7. Literate in primary language: yes ☐   no ☐

VII. Vocational Status

1. Vocational history for past 10 years:

   Employer:_____

   From:_____to:_____

Position/occupation:_____

Job duties:_____

Wage:_____

Reason for leaving:_____

2. Vocational/educational goals:_____

3. Amount of compensation benefits:_____

VIII. Results of Physician Interview

1. Name:_____　　Phone:_____

   Specialty: _____

2. Diagnosis:_____

3. Prognosis:_____

4. Treatment plan:_____

5. Time frames:_____

6. Projected return-to-work date

   Light duty:_____　　Regular duty:_____

7. Planned surgeries:_____

   Anticipated hospital length of stay:_____

   Postsurgery treatment and time frames:_____

8. Possible complications:_____

IX. Results of Employer Interview

1. Name:_____　　Position:_____

2. Length of employment:_____

3. Position:_____

4. Job duties:_____

_____

5. Is client required to do the following:

	Percent of day
Lifting	_____
Bending	_____
Carrying	_____
Sitting	_____
Standing	_____
Climbing	_____
Driving	_____
Crawling	_____
Repetitive tasks	_____

6. Approximately how many pounds is the client required to lift/ carry, etc: _____

7. Does client have special training: yes ☐   no ☐

8. Are other positions available for the client: yes ☐   no ☐

9. Light-duty availability:_____

10. Comments:_____

11. Is client considered a motivated employee: yes ☐   no ☐

12. Is there any additional information you believe is relevant?

_____
_____
_____

X. Case Manager's Opinions/Impressions

_____
_____
_____
_____

XI. Case Manager's Recommendations

_____
_____
_____
_____

XII. Projected Costs

_____
_____

Table 4-2. Initial Assessment Tool for a Client with Health Insurance

Name:_____	Referral source:_____
Insured:_____	Address:_____
Policy #:_____	_____
Social Security #:_____	_____
Address:_____	_____
Phone:_____	Phone:_____ Fax:_____
	Contact person:_____
Date of birth:_____	Date of diagnosis:_____
Diagnosis:_____	

Type of insurance: Managed care:_____ Specific type:_____

Indemnity:_____ Group:_____ Individual:_____

Self-insured:_____ Medicare:____ Medicaid:_____

I. Introduction

1. Reason for referral:_____

2. Place of interview/parties present: _____

3. Employer:_____

   Address:_____

   _____

   Phone:_____ Fax:_____

   Contact person:_____

II. History of Illness

Date diagnosed:_____

III. Current Status

1. Height:_____ Weight:_____ Premorbid weight:_____

2. Systems review

   Overall appearance

   Skin Integrity

     Problems:_____

     Treatment:_____

     Outcome:_____

   Sensory/neurological status

     Problems:_____

     Treatment:_____

     Outcome:_____

   Nutritional status

     Problems:_____

     Treatment:_____

     Outcome:_____

   Gastrointestinal status

     Problems:_____

     Treatment:_____

     Outcome:_____

Genitourinary status
   Problems:_____
   Treatment:_____
   Outcome:_____
Cardiovascular status
   Problems:_____
   Treatment:_____
   Outcome:_____
Respiratory status
   Problems:_____
   Treatment:_____
   Outcome:_____
Musculoskeletal status
   Problems:_____
   Treatment:_____
   Outcome:_____
Endocrine status
   Problems:_____
   Treatment:_____
   Outcome:_____
Immunological status
   Problems:_____
   Treatment:_____
   Outcome:_____
3. Medication:_____
4. Functional abilities:

Self-care	Independent	Min. assist	Mod. assist	Totally dependent
Hygiene	☐	☐	☐	☐
Toileting	☐	☐	☐	☐
Dressing	☐	☐	☐	☐
Eating	☐	☐	☐	☐
Food prep	☐	☐	☐	☐
Transportation	☐	☐	☐	☐
Ambulation	☐	☐	☐	☐

5. Subjective complaints:_____

6. Objective data:_____

7. Equipment/supplies:_____

8. Home care:_____

9. Providers:

    a. Physician

        Name:_____   Specialty:_____

        Address:_____

        _____

        Phone:_____   Fax:_____

III. Medical History

1. Previous hospitalizations (dates, treatments):_____

    _____

2. Past serious illnesses/injuries:_____

    _____

IV. Psychosocial Status

1. Marital status:_____

    Spouse's occupation/hours at work:_____

    _____

2. Dependents (number, ages):_____

    _____

3. Caregiver/support system: _____

    _____

4. Home environment:

    Lives with:_____

    Barriers:_____

    _____

    Status of neighborhood:_____

    Community resources:_____

V. Educational/Vocational Status

1. Occupation:_____

2. Job duties:_____

3. Currently working: yes ☐   no ☐

4. Return-to-work projections: _____

VI. Result of Physician Interview

Name:_____   Specialty:_____

Phone:_____

Diagnosis:_____

Prognosis:_____

Treatment plan:_____

Expected/projected complications:_____

VII. Opinions/Impressions/Recommendations

_____

_____

_____

_____

VIII. Projected Costs

_____

_____

_____

In the course of data collection, conflicting or contradictory information may surface. It is the role of the nurse case manager to gather additional information, inform all members of the health care team what the data revealed, and work toward conflict resolution if necessary.

Where the assessment is performed depends upon the case manager's place of employment. The case manager in the acute care facility will perform the initial assessment immediately prior to admission or, at the latest, very shortly after the patient's admission to the hospital. The case manager working for an insurance carrier will perform an assessment either by telephone (referred to as "telephonic case management" by people in the industry) or on-site. The on-site assessment can be in the person's home, at a physician's office before or after a scheduled appointment, or in the acute care facility, rehabilitation institute, or subacute unit. Because the home environment is a crucial piece in the assessment process, a home visit, where the client is apt to be more relaxed, is the most desirable and will result in the most comprehensive assessment. Telephonic assessments yield the least comprehensive results.

Unless incapable of communicating, the client is the primary source of information in the assessment process. Family members and/or the client's support system are secondary providers of information. Additional data are collected through review of the medical records and collaboration with all health care providers. Depending on the specific diagnosis or place of injury, the client's employer is often an additional source of information. In workers' compensation injuries, the employer plays a large part in the assessment process. A complete vocational and educational history is critical to assist the client to return to work. This aspect of case management will be dealt with in more depth in Chapter 7.

PERSONAL SKILLS

Organization and Time Management

A comprehensive assessment should take between 1 and 2 hours. If the interview lasts more than 2 hours, the nurse case manager may not be reimbursed for the time. It is important to remember that the referral source and/or insurance carriers often put time limits on various parts of the case management process. The case manager's ability to meet the goals depends in part on organizational skills and effective use of time. Time management skills and organizational skills work together. If the case manager is disorganized or easily distracted, and/or allows other team members to become distracted, the focus will be lost, time will be wasted, and the case management process will fail.

The case manager must be aware of treatment plans and recommended time frames. Positive outcomes of critical pathways depend on accomplishing various aspects of care along a timeline. The LAMP method will assist the case manager in maintaining time effectiveness and organization:

*L*ist essential things to complete each day, in order of priority.

*A*ccurate record keeping will avoid delays in treatment or outcomes.

*M*aximize the use of voice mail by leaving and requesting detailed
messages.

*P*hone calls should be short and succinct.

The case manager must use the telephone efficiently. Often a complete plan of care can be implemented through effective use of a fax
machine and voice mail. If the case manager leaves a detailed message, rather than a request for a return call, the receiver can begin
responding immediately.

Prioritization

The ability to prioritize is an intrinsic component of organizational
skill and time management. Within any aspect of health care the emergency is often the rule, not the exception. The nurse case manager
must have the skills to give the unforeseen priority at a moment's
notice. Excellent organizational skills won't bail out an inflexible
person, one who finds it so difficult to rearrange her or his daily list
of activities that urgent issues are not dealt with expeditiously. The
result is a breakdown of the system. Differentiating among urgent,
important, and minor distinguishes successful case management
from mediocre care.

Establishing priorities requires well-defined objectives. The
nurse case manager who does not have clearly defined goals and
objectives will be unable to set priorities. What may be considered
urgent under one circumstance may be minor in another situation.
Knowing what the goals are will allow for ease in determining what
is important in a specific situation.

For example, a nurse case manager works with a hospitalized,
elderly client whose diagnosis is cellulitis of the left lower extremity. She is debilitated with mild COPD and has right hemiplegia as a
result of a CVA 2 years ago. The client lives in a rural area with
her adult son, who is employed as a salesman for a large corporation.

The discharge plan includes the following: fully electric hospital bed; commode with removable arms; home health aide 8 hours daily, 5 days per week; IV antibiotic therapy; physical therapist to teach home health aide and client's son range-of-motion exercises. The nurse case manager receives authorization from the insurance carrier to coordinate and implement the discharge plan.

The nurse case manager needs to prioritize the order in which he or she implements the home care. The first priority would be to coordinate the services of the home health aide, since that is the most difficult piece to put in place. It can often take 24 to 48 hours or more to coordinate appropriate home care. Since the client lives in a rural area, finding appropriate care may take even longer. The second piece of the discharge plan that the case manager would coordinate is the IV therapy. The physician must be contacted to obtain the prescription, which is faxed to the IV company. The IV company would follow up by coordinating the required skilled nursing visits for the antibiotic infusions and delivery of all the necessary equipment and supplies. The third piece that the nurse case manager would coordinate is delivery of the hospital bed and commode. The physical therapy visit is the last service to be coordinated. If the case manager needs an additional day or two to coordinate a therapy visit, the client's discharge would not be delayed.

Prioritizing is continuous. The case manager's list of priorities can change from moment to moment throughout the day. Many times different members of the health care team will feel their treatment recommendation is of higher priority than someone else's. It is the case manager's job to rank priorities for the client appropriately and swiftly without offending or minimizing the other team member's requests.

Delegation

An important tool in organization and time management is delegating. "Delegation is defined as sharing responsibility and authority with subordinates and holding them accountable for performance."[23]

Delegating is different from directing. *Directing* involves showing someone how to do something. *Delegating* is giving a person who is competent a task to do and expecting the task will be completed. To delegate is not to give up control nor is it to shirk one's responsibilities. Rather, it is through effective delegation of tasks that goals will be achieved and positive outcomes will be realized.

Most nurse case managers with large caseloads cannot accomplish all the desired objectives efficiently if they feel that they have to "do it all." A belief in the adage "if you want something done correctly, do it yourself" interferes with the case manager's ability to delegate. The result is noncompletion of objectives, delay in coordination of care, increased risk of complications, and increased cost of care. Delegating, a byproduct of leadership skills, ensures that the objectives are met in order of priority and in a timely manner.

The case manager is a facilitator, responsible for coordinating or delegating care to specialists in various fields. If the client with diabetes needs nutritional counseling, the nurse case manager should delegate that aspect of care to a dietitian or nutritionist. The case manager who is tempted to do the teaching herself or himself is not using time efficiently.

Creativity

Much of the case management process involves utilizing resources in an original manner. Along with a broad and comprehensive knowledge base, the nurse case manager should be a creative thinker. Problem solving and critical thinking involve flexibility and creativity. In today's rapidly shifting health care arena, the nurse case manager who is a creative thinker will have the ability to keep pace.

Self-Discipline

Many nurse case managers work independently and autonomously. Many external nurse case managers work from their homes. Self-discipline, initiative, and self-direction are essential traits of the successful nurse case manager. The experienced case manager receives little direction, has flexibility in scheduling appointments, and does not often need to account for his or her time. The nurse case manager without self-discipline and self-direction may delay coordination of care at the expense of the client, the insurance carrier, the physician, and all other members of the multidisciplinary health care team. If the nurse case manager procrastinates, the finely tuned system of collaborative, high-quality, and cost-effective care will crumble.

Chapter Highlights

* Nurse case managers must possess a broad range of skills to achieve positive outcomes from the case management process.
* For the purpose of organization we have classified the required skills into four basic categories, although the elements will overlap at times.
* Interpersonal skills include: communication, both verbal and written; tact and diplomacy; assertiveness; collaboration and negotiation.
* Professional skills include: marketing, negotiation, and investigation.
* Knowledge-based skills include: critical thinking and problem solving research, and assessment.
* Personal skills include: organization and time management; prioritization; delegation; creativity, and self-discipline.

References

1.   Clark, M. (1992). *Nursing in the community*. Norwalk, CT: Appleton & Lange. p. 283.
2.   Ibid., pp. 283–295.
3.   Ibid., p. 301.
4.   Ibid., p. 302.
5.   Pear, R. (1995/Dec. 21). Doctors say HMOs limit what they can tell patients. *New York Times*. p. 1.

6. Arnold, E., & Boggs, K. (1989). *Interpersonal relationships: professional communication skills for nurses*. Philadelphia, PA: W.B. Saunders. p. 360.

7. Hein, E., & Nicholson, J. (1986). *Contemporary leadership behavior: Selected readings* (2d ed.). Boston, MA: Little, Brown. p. 121.

8. Arnold & Boggs, *Interpersonal relationships*. p. 361.

9. Ibid., p. 392.

10. Sullivan, E., & Decker, P. (1988). *Effective management in nursing* (2d ed.). Menlo Park, CA: Addison-Wesley. p. 566.

11. St. Coeur, M., & Steinberg, A. (1996). *Case management practice guidelines*. St. Louis, MO: Mosby. p. 16.

12. International Association of Special Investigation Units. (1995/May 10). National Insurance Fraud Forum white paper. p. viii.

13. Sullivan & Decker, *Effective management in nursing*. p. 263.

14. Ibid.

15. Ibid., p. 264.

16. Ibid.

17. Ibid., pp. 265–270.

18. Cohen, E., & Cesta, T. (1993). *Nursing case management from concept to evolution*. St. Louis, MO: Mosby. p. 130.

19. Potter, P., & Perry, A. (1993). *Fundamentals of nursing: concepts, process & practice* (3d ed.). St Louis, MO: Mosby. p. 236.

20. Ibid., p. 237.

21. Ibid., p. 238.

22. Treece, E., & Treece, J. (1977). *Elements of research nursing* (2d ed.). St Louis, MO: Mosby. p. 47.

23. Sullivan & Decker, *Effective management in nursing*. p. 251.

Internal Case 5
Management

Nurse case managers working within health care facilities are referred to as "internal" case managers. Internal case management began in the acute care setting as a result of hospital restructuring to provide less costly care, standardize treatments, and improve quality. As the goals of case management expanded to include coordination of care across the continuum, internal case management began to flourish in settings other than the acute care hospitals. Today, internal case managers are found in acute care facilities, rehabilitation institutes, subacute facilities, and home care agencies.

This chapter explores the evolution of the role of the internal case manager in various settings. Upon completion of this chapter you will be able to answer the following questions:

1. How did the role of the case manager evolve in the acute care setting?
2. What models of case management are currently being used in the acute care setting?
3. How do critical pathways guide the process of case management?
4. How does the setting of client care (acute care versus community-based versus rehabilitation versus subacute versus home care) influence the role of the case manager?

OVERVIEW

When reviewing the literature, you will realize that a multitude of case management models are described. Depending on the definition used for the term *model*, you will find descriptions based on different foci. You will find models differentiated by disease entities, by setting, by the educational background of the case manager, and by the uniqueness of the institution in which it is practiced. You will also find that a particular model may be referred to by several different names in various journals or books.

To organize and simplify the structure of case management, we describe case management according to setting: institutional-based case management, community-based case management, and insurance-based case management. It is interesting that institutional case management and insurance case management have evolved with separate yet parallel histories.

Insurance case management (also referred to as "external" case management), which will be discussed in depth in Chapter 6, evolved in the 1970s as an outgrowth of high dollar claims. As case management began to reduce the cost of health care delivery, independent case management firms began to grow in the private sector. Today, external case managers are working in the insurance industry as employees of insurance companies or as independent contractors and in home care agencies.

THE ACUTE CARE SETTING

An acute care setting is an "institution for treatment of the sick and injured."[1] It is estimated that there are approximately 6600 acute care hospitals in the United States. Because of the rapidly shifting health care and economic environments, many services previously requiring hospitalization are now performed in ambulatory settings, subacute facilities, or in the home. This shift has decreased occupied hospital beds, which translates into a loss of generated income. In addition, budget cuts have threatened to close many city hospitals.

Many acute care facilities have been forced to close, to merge with other institutions, or to develop alternative health care product lines such as primary care services.

The most recent statistics available, from 1993, show a stated average patient stay in the acute care facility of 7.0 days. The average cost to hospitals per patient day is $880.52. The average cost to hospitals per patient stay is $6,132.06.[2] These statistics are based on a national average.

Until the 1980s, the focus of health care in this country was on increasing technology. Hospitals proliferated, the physician-patient ratio decreased, and the cost of health care rose at an alarming rate. By the middle of the decade, it became evident that if the system were allowed to continue on its present course, the number of uninsured and underinsured people would continue to escalate and limit appropriate care to a small group of rich elite. Available health care resources would diminish and eventually lead to a deterioration in the total health care delivery system. Cost containment practices had to be put in place. The focus of health care delivery shifted from "high tech to high speed."[3] The growth of managed care organizations has promoted a shift from specialist to generalist; from performing tasks to cost accountability; from treatment to prevention.

As a result of the changes in health care, the role of the nurse has been redefined to include fiscal responsibility. Since nursing is a 24-hour phenomenon, the nurse can control much of the use of hospital resources. The nurse case manager in the acute care setting is an outgrowth of cost containment practices. The case manager role has been further supported by the autonomy and professionalism nursing has achieved since the 1970s. Internal, or institution-based, case management began in the acute care setting in 1985. As institutional case management became entrenched in the acute care hospitals, models of case management were designed to incorporate differences unique to each setting. As the emphasis of case management shifted from solely cost savings to include increased quality of care across the continuum, institutional case management emerged in rehabilitation and subacute facilities, as well as in hospital-affiliated home care agencies.

(see Figure 5-1). At this time, nursing case management is used in many institutions to increase quality, decrease fragmentation of care, decrease the cost of care, and maximize utilization of resources.

EARLY MODELS OF CASE MANAGEMENT IN ACUTE CARE

As an outgrowth of primary nursing and of the emergence of diagnosis-related groups (DRGs) in 1983, case management found its way into the acute care setting. For the first time, health care providers had limitations placed on hospital length of stay and on their use of resources. The DRG is a complex classification system "of client diagnoses for which typical costs of care have been calculated, based on the cost of specific services required."[4] The federal government initiated use of the DRG system to reimburse hospitals for services provided under Medicare. This established prospective payment to hospitals. There are currently 467 DRGs. Each DRG is based upon a specific illness category, diagnosis, and expected length of stay. For example, if a patient is admitted for chemotherapy, the allowed hospitalization is 2.6 days. If the patient is discharged after 1 day, the hospital's profit increases. If the patient is discharged after 3 days, the hospital loses money.

When these limitations became a reality, acute care facilities needed to rethink their methods of care delivery. In the past, hospitals charged a per diem rate based upon their costs. In that type of reimbursement system, there was no motivation to practice economically, because all costs of delivering care could be billed to the patient and reimbursed by the insurer. However, with fixed, prospective reimbursement, achieving outcomes that could be measured within a predetermined time frame became a necessity.

Many acute care facilities began to redefine their methods using terminology and practices from private industry. Increasing productivity, increasing profits, and decreasing losses were translated into providing continuity of care, decreasing fragmentation and duplication of services to maximize the utilization of resources.

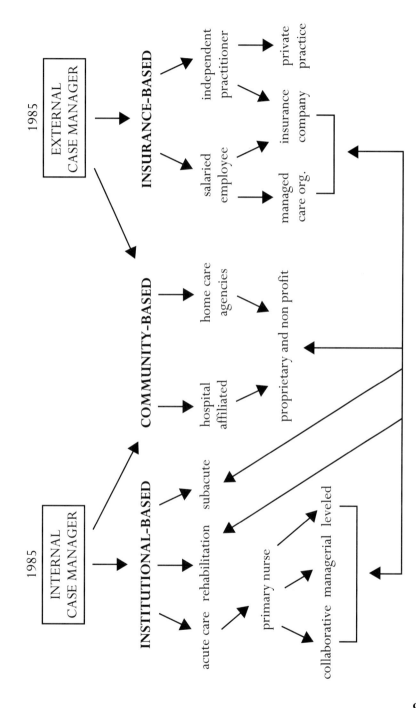

Figure 5-1. *Nurse case management models*

95

The New England Medical Center Hospital Model

One of the earliest case management programs in acute care was formulated in 1985, at the New England Medical Center Hospital (NEMCH) in Boston, Massachusetts, under the development of Karen Zander, RN, MS, CS. This model has also been referred to as the *New England Medical Center Nursing Model*; the *North Eastern Model*, and the *Primary Nurse Model*. The goal was to decrease hospital length of stay without compromising quality of care. The objective was to find a positive balance among cost, quality, and the process of care.

Zander's triad

Zander saw this restructuring as a means of advancing the nursing profession and redefining the role of the bedside nurse. In transforming patient care to fit a managed care environment, the model applied a systems framework which considered structure, process, and outcome, linked by the triad of design, role, and feedback (see Figure 5-2). *Design* is application of the nursing process. *Role* is the primary nurse, or case manager, and *feedback* is the information necessary for revisions, or the evaluation process. Evaluation of outcomes can be either concurrent or retrospective. *Concurrent review* takes place during the patient's hospitalization as a means of prob-

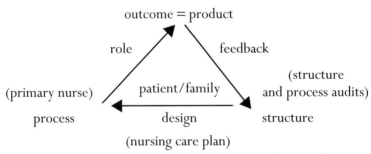

Figure 5-2.   *NEMCH case management model.* (Adapted from Zander, K., Etheredge, M., & Bower, K. (1987). *Nursing case management: blueprint for transformation.* Waban, MA.: Winslow, p. 3)

lem identification. *Retrospective review* takes place on the day of discharge, or after, to assess trends.

Zander based her model on five beliefs, or assumptions, shown in Table 5-1.

Zander discusses the development of primary nursing in a three-generation construct, over the past 90 years: the preprimary

Table 5-1. Assumption of the New England Medical Center Nursing Model

1. Nurses have always been managers of care but have labored with outdated management tools (such as nursing care plans) and shift-centered management systems.

2. Quality is not a vague ideal but rather is definable using specific clinical process amd outcome standards that are the resolution of patient problems. Quality in health care is thus a product, not a service.

3. The true cost of producing a range of expected outcomes can be understood and revised on a case-type basis. Diagnostic related groups (DRGs) are not in themselves descriptive of costs because they are based on a biomedical model. On the other hand, the more (potentially) controllable costs of an episode of care are in the nursing realm of self-care deficits and physical complications (respiratory, immobility, etc.) that can often be prevented through astute management.

4. Nursing makes a major contribution to clinical outcomes through powerful interventions based on a diagnostic reasoning process and by making the system work for the physicans and patients. Because of nursing's 24-hour access, nursing allocates much of a hospital's resources.

5. Nurses and physicians have always worked interdependently, but in parallel structures rather than in formal collaborative practice groups with protocols. Also, clinicians tend to assume that high technical know-how indicates high case management skills, which is not necessarily true. Therefore, even highly skilled clinicians can benefit from learning updated management strategies.[5]

generation was highly centralized, task-oriented, and physician-controlled. With the first generation of primary nursing, the role of the nurse was expanded from doer to thinker. The nurse was seen as an expert in her or his own right and not as an extension of the physician. During the second generation of primary nursing, nursing became decentralized. Nurses and physicians collaborated to make mutually agreeable decisions. The nurse was given the "locus of accountability." (See Table 5-2).

It was during the second generation of primary nursing that case management in the acute care facility became a reality. After a 2-year investigation of nursing and physician practices at The New England Medical Center Hospital, a group of primary nurses was chosen to take on the role of case manager. Before beginning, they were given extra training in management.

The primary nurse assumed a higher level of authority than he or she had traditionally. The primary nurse's new role was no longer merely to coordinate services; by applying clinical judgment, the nurse began to organize and evaluate services, with the authority to ensure compliance of the plan.

Nursing was further enhanced by empowering the nurse to "hold the locus of accountability."[6] This means that the primary nurse who has determined what patient outcomes are expected is held answerable for whether the outcomes are achieved, regardless of which personnel actually delivered the patient care. Zander differentiates between accountability and responsibility. All staff nurses are responsible. Accountability, however, is determined through achieving predefined results, which are the desired outcomes.

As an example, consider the nurse teaching self-injection to a newly diagnosed client with diabetes. The desired outcome is successful self-injection. How this is taught or by whom is not evaluated; rather, the patient's ability and accuracy in self-injecting is the accountable outcome. The primary nurse's or case manager's accountability is measured by that successful outcome. The actual patient teaching can be performed by any staff nurse.

Zander stresses that 24-hour accountability is not synonymous with 24-hour availability. She argues that when a nurse is on call 24

Table 5-2. Developmental Stages of Professional Practice

Components	1900–1969: Pre-Primary Nursing	Transition	1969–1985: First-Generation Primary Nursing	Transition	1985–1995: Second-Generation Nursing/Case Management
Focal point	Tasks with responsibility		Process with individuality		Outcomes (product) accountability
Power base	Dependent on extension of MD's expert and legitimate power	Parallelism	RN as expert	Collaborative practice with MDs, peers, and system	Referent power is shared goals
Role and identity	Doer; reporter	Care planner	Thinker, therapeutic nurse-patient relationship which includes families	Patient-teacher	Case manager→Healer
Evaluation	Personal qualities & completion of responsibilities	Overall behavioral objectives for RNs	Competence	Outcome standards per patient; process standards for nurse	Effectiveness (within quality standards)
Quality assurance	Problem identification	Target, anonymous audits	Nursing process	Comprehensive, personal & system audits (e.g., MIS)	Nursing product
Staff/unit organization	8-hr (shift) focus; use of team, functional, total patient care; interchangeable staff. Continuity sporadic	End of shift "kingdoms"; continuity methods. Assignments of PN to patient	24-hr focus per patient per primary nurse; use of geographic, modular & other case assignment methods. LPN's, RN's, PN→Aides	Flextime; formal associates	Length of stay focus per patient per primary nurse across episode of care: Use of continuous & collaborative professional practice groups. PN/CM LPNs, Aides RN's, Other Disciplines MD
Management structures & processes	Highly centralized; attention to rules	Head nurse as manager	Decentralized; attention to group dynamics; staff nurses' clinical decision making & coordination	Staff nurse as manager	Mix of centralized & decentralized; attention to organization and system
Skills	"Instrumental functions," Bureaucratic; rule-passing	BSN	"Expressive functions," participative interactions	BSN/MSN: inquiry; nurse-to-nurse learning	Group membership & leadership Management skills Clinical research consultation Contracting

Copyright, NEMCH, 1985. Developed by K. Zander. Reprinted with permission.

hours per day, it may signal possessiveness and overinvolvement in the patient's care on the part of the nurse, a scenario fostered by many primary nursing systems. This would compromise, not improve, communication, collaboration, and management.

In the past, the product of the acute care system was nursing care. Zander redefined the product to equate with outcomes, which are observable, measurable, and directly related to cost. Nursing care becomes the process for achieving these outcomes, and the primary nurse, or case manager, is the person accountable for achieving positive outcomes. Zander defines case management as the "production process."[7] She further elaborates by describing case management as "cutting across hierarchical lines to produce a closed loop process."[8] Others have described case management as establishing a "seamless operation." Simply stated, case management is a system created to fill the gaps created by a fragmented health care delivery system, and to accomplish this in a cost-effective, time-efficient manner, across the entire continuum of care.

The development of critical pathways

The New England Medical Center Model of case management has four components: (1) achievement of outcomes; (2) the case manager as caregiver; (3) nurse/physician group practices; and (4) active participation by the client system.[9]

Until now, nursing care plans were used as the guide for nursing care. In reality, the care plans were rarely referred to, were seldom updated, were never formed from a multidisciplinary effort, and were not developed according to a predetermined length of stay. A tool was needed that would incorporate a multidisciplinary, proactive approach to a collaborative provider environment, with DRG-allotted time as the guide. Thus, the nursing staff at the New England Medical Center Hospital developed case management plans that kept in mind the goal of decreasing cost and maintaining quality.

Each case management plan was designed by case type (DRG), rather than for each individual patient, and outlined detailed, day-by-day nursing practice. The plan included projected utilization of resources and patient outcomes, related to a specific diagnosis. The patient outcomes were reviewed and agreed to by physicians and nurses. The plan was later abbreviated and condensed to 1 page of information called a "critical pathway."

A *critical pathway*, also referred to as a *clinical pathway* or a *multidisciplinary action plan (MAP)* is defined as "the critical or key events expected to happen each day of a patient's hospitalization."[10] When designing a critical pathway, the DRG is used as a guide in determining the length of stay. The critical pathway, like the case management plan, is also developed by case type. It is a grid outlining treatment along a timeline with expected outcomes. Categories listed in the critical pathway include, but are not limited to assessment and evaluation, tests, consults, activity, treatments, medications, diet, teaching, and discharge planning.

Timelines are essential in the development of the critical pathway. A timeline is a specified period over which an event is expected to occur. Timelines can be measured in hours or minutes, as in the emergency room; in days or weeks, which are typically used for diagnoses with clear expectations of length of stay, such as "abdominal pain/rule out appendicitis"; or in months, as in the neonatal intensive care units or long-term care facilities.

The case manager maintains control by continuously assessing whether the client is meeting the expected critical pathway outcomes. If the outcome is not achieved, the case manager documents this as a variance. A variance is any outcome that has not been achieved. A variance is the result of any one of four circumstances: system or operational; provider; patient; or unmet clinical indicators. (See Table 5-3.)

The critical pathway, in conjunction with interdisciplinary meetings, is used by the case manager in coordinating, monitoring, and evaluating patient care. The nurse case manager uses the critical pathway both as a tool for early identification of problems—to assess if the problem is nursing-related, patient-related, or hospital-related—and as a guide to eliminate unnecessary procedures and delays in discharge. The critical pathway can be used in conjunction with nursing care plans. The focus is to achieve desired patient outcomes within predetermined and specific time frames. Critical pathways have succeeded in standardizing treatment and evaluating outcomes because they were relatively easy to develop and lack abstract terminology.

Critical pathways do not compromise quality in the name of cost savings. Rather, cost containment is realized through minimizing variation in clinical outcomes, quantifying quality, and enhancing

Table 5-3. Examples of the Four Types of Outcome Variances

System or Operational Variance Examples

Broken equipment

Lost requisition slips causing delays

Departmental delays due to staffing or other causes

Interdepartmental delays

Larger system delays affecting discharge, such as home care services, equipment, or insurance availability

Health Care Provider Variance Examples

Deviation from plan due to physician varying the practice pattern

Change related to health care provider's practice patterns, level of expertise, or experience

Patient Variance Examples

Refusal	Change in status	Unavailability

Unmet Clinical Quality Examples

Intermediate outcomes:

    Patient is off IV Solumedrol when peak flow > 200

    Discharge outcomes:

    Peak flow measurement > 250 L/sec

    Patient is out of bed without shortness of breath

Patient is able to return demonstration of the use of MDI with spacer

Source: Adapted from E. Cohen & T. Cesta, (1993), *Nursing case management: From concept to evaluation*. St. Louis: Mosby, pp. 123–124) with permission.

collaboration of services. Timely treatment is obviously of great importance in generating cost savings. Case management in conjunction with critical pathways can ensure consistency and continuity of care and eliminate duplication or fragmentation of services that is common in many large medical centers.

From the evolution of the critical pathway, Zander developed a more elaborate tool, the *CareMap*. Referred to as the "second generation" of critical pathways, the CareMap expands the focus of intervention to include problem statements, intermediate goals, and outcomes.[11] It is described as "a cause and effect grid which identifies expected patient and/or family and staff behaviors against a timeline for a case type or otherwise defined homogeneous population. The four essential parts of a CareMap tool are a timeline, an index of problems with intermediate and outcome criteria, a critical path, and a variance record."[12] The CareMap is based on the premise that daily actions of the staff will cause certain reactions or responses from the patient and/or family, which over time become the desired outcomes. Actions by the staff are referred to as "standards of practice," and the patient and family responses, which are predictable among homogeneous populations, describe "standards of care."[13]

In many institutions the critical pathway remains part of the medical record and incorporates the necessary criteria that the Joint Commission on Accreditation of Health Care Organizations (JCAHO) requires. As of 1994, JCAHO required a multidisciplinary, collaborative approach to health care delivery that includes mechanisms to measure improvement of performance and quality of care.

Because of differences within settings, the terminology used when referring to critical pathways can be confusing and often overlapping. Some facilities differentiate between a critical pathway and a MAP, other settings use the terms synonymously, and some institutions combine the terms and develop a form unique to that facility. For simplicity, we are using the terms *critical pathway*, *clinical pathway*, *CareMap* and *MAP* to describe a detailed plan outlining treatment—based on diagnosis with expected outcomes along a timeline. Through appropriate use of the critical pathway the providers of care can determine the variances that are delaying the desired outcomes. The case manager in collaboration with the multidisciplinary team can then focus treatment around the variances.

In Zander's model, the patient is assigned to a group of nurses and a physician at or before admission. A primary nurse is chosen, who becomes the case manager and is accountable clinically and financially throughout the patient's hospital stay. Prior to admission the nurse case manager contacts the patient at home, to orient the patient to the anticipated care. The case manager also takes a thorough health history to uncover any existing problems or needs that could extend the hospitalization or necessitate individualization of critical paths.[14] Discharge planning is outlined before admission, with changes made as needed after admission.

While the patient is in the unit, the nurse case manager is the primary caregiver and continues to coordinate, direct, and monitor care as the patient is moved throughout the hospital. Regular team meetings allow for necessary changes in treatment and for problem solving. These meetings include the nursing group and the physician.

Outcomes of the NEMCH model

This model was first tested on clients with two types of diagnoses: stroke and leukemia (in adults). In one study, outcomes were reviewed after 6 months for those patients admitted with ischemic stroke. It was found that with the nurse case management model, there was a 29 percent drop in the average length of stay and a 47 percent drop in the average number of days spent in the intensive care unit.[15] The results from the group with leukemia were just as impressive. Patient hospitalization was decreased by approximately 10 to 15 days, through a reduction in unnecessary diagnostic testing and coordination of chemotherapy to be infused at home. In addition, increased patient satisfaction resulted—patients felt they had more control over their care, and infection rates decreased, indicating higher quality of care. From these successes, the case management process was expanded to include additional diagnoses.[16]

Today, the case management program at New England Medical Center Hospital has been modified to fit the rapidly changing health care environment. Hospital restructuring, downsizing, and overlapping of roles, in addition to the ubiquitous infiltration of managed care, has forced the creation of two systems of case management. Clinical case management accounts for approximately 40 percent of the clients receiving case management, and the other 60 percent involve *utilization review*. Most acute care facilities have a utilization review department, staffed by nurses who determine the necessity and appropriateness of medical services. Included is review of length of stay and discharge plans.

The shift in health care practice, and the conversion of patient homes into "minihospitals," has changed the scope of case management. The focus today is to identify which population is best served through a case management model. And the role of the case manager has been redefined as either "episode-based" or "continuum-based." *Episode-based* case management takes place within a specific time frame, such as one hospitalization stay, and ends at discharge. In *continuum-based* case management, the process continues beyond discharge, for an indefinite period of time or until there is a resolution of issues.[17]

It is generally agreed that 20 percent or less of the patient population benefits significantly from case management. In choosing an appropriate selection measure, Zander differentiates between *acuity* and *complexity*. The patient with an acute problem, such as an episode of angina requiring hospitalization, may or may not benefit from case management. The elderly patient with varied health problems, requiring the utilization of multiple resources, presents a complexity of issues that would definitely require case management involvement.

In addition, research by Stetler and DeZell showed that the high cost of acute care can be attributed to four problem areas that must be included in the planning and designing of case management programs for the catastrophically ill population. These four are:

1. *Potential for complications—self-care*: Presence of risk factors that may limit a patient's ability to manage his or her own disease and/or engage in health-promoting activities in the home environment.

2. *Potential for injury unrelated to treatment:* Presence of risk factors related primarily to the person's general state of health, and/or to specific disease symptoms that could lead to physical injury within the institutional setting.

3. *Potential for complications related to treatment:* Presence of risk factors, at times inherent in the in-hospital treatment, that endanger the health and safety of the patient if (a) appropriate preventive measures are not instituted and maintained and/or (b) ongoing observations and monitoring are not instituted.

4. *Potential for extension of the disease process:* Presence of a specific condition or pathological process that carries with it a risk that endangers the recovery of the patient, i.e., presence of a risk that will be increased if a treatable extension or sequelae are undetected.[18]

Zander's proposed system of case management has been incorporated into several other acute care facilities, with modifications to fit the individual philosophies, budgets, and nursing resources of the institution. Two examples follow of how the basic concept of primary nurse as case manager was altered to fit a specific institution.

Case Management at St. Michael Hospital

In 1988, St. Michael Hospital in Milwaukee, Wisconsin, introduced a case management program based on the New England Medical Center model. A few minor adaptations were necessary to fit the model to the institution, including expansion of the critical pathway and specific interventions to encourage physician collaboration. Two categories were added to the critical pathway: key nursing activities/teaching, and key patient activities/outcomes. A section for professional review organization (PRO) discharge screens was also added.[19] *Discharge screens* are developed upon admission to document criteria that should be met upon discharge. If these criteria are not met, a peer review organization looks at the treatment and variances to determine unresolved problems and issues.[20]

Other modifications to the New England Medical Center model include totally unit-based case management. When the patient is moved from unit to unit, the case management process is transferred to the case manager on the new unit.

Case Management at Hillcrest Medical Center

Hillcrest Medical Center in Tulsa, Oklahoma, a 646-bed acute care facility, also incorporated the New England Medical Center model into its design. A system of selecting DRGs that would benefit from case management was established. Major diagnostic categories were analyzed according to volume, profitability, and financial trends. The categories with the highest patient volume and lowest profit margin were chosen for case management. Following implementation of case management, data showed that approximately "$960,000 of billed charges and 430 patient days were saved through nursing case management."[21]

Alternate Approaches to Acute Care Case Management

With the growing emphasis on controlling the cost of health care, and the explosion of managed care, case management within the acute care setting continues to evolve. Decreased length of hospital stay, lower RN-to-nonprofessional-staff ratio, and the changing role of the primary nurse led to modification of the case management model originally used at the New England Medical Center Hospital. Two more ways that other acute-care facilities incorporate case management into their systems, using different methods of achieving positive outcomes, can be grouped as (1) *leveled case management*, in which the nurse case manager is at least baccalaureate-prepared and does not deliver direct patient care; and (2) *managerial* or *collaborative case management*, where the nurse case manager, a part of a multidisciplinary group, has increased fiscal and management responsibilities.

Leveled case management

In 1987, Sharp Memorial Hospital in San Diego developed leveled case management. The concept of a professional and technical nursing practice model had previously been tested in two successful pilot programs at Yale-New Haven Hospital in 1986.[22] Sharp Memorial Hospital based its leveled case management program on the success of the Yale-New Haven project.[23] The nursing administrators believed that although primary nursing was still a valued philosophy of delivery of care, its emphasis had been on implementing and evaluating a plan of care, rather than managing that care. It was found that the primary nursing model of case management was not effective in "bridging financial and quality of care issues brought on by cost containment measures of the 1980s."[24] When the direct caregiver is also the case manager, management needs may become compromised when patient care is the main priority.

As with Zander, the administrators at Sharp Memorial adapted management philosophies from private industry. The theme was based on providing efficient service through coordination of care across departments and disciplines. In addition, downsizing eliminated middle management, resulting in authority trickling down to the lowest levels.

The three issues that needed to be addressed in redesigning the organizational structure were to define the role of the case manager, to clarify the definition of caseload, (either by DRG, physician, or unit) to design a tool to monitor operations on specific units, and to evaluate the impact of case management on the hospital.

The case management system that evolved defined both a professional and a technical level of nursing. The professional level required the nurse to have a baccalaureate degree; the technical level required an associate degree. In this program, the professional nurse is the case manager. Her or his responsibilities include managing clinical care, determining outcomes, and facilitating the achievement of those outcomes. Direct patient care is provided by the technical level nurse and nursing assistants.

Caseload was defined by the physician, mainly because only a few physicians accounted for the majority of admissions. These physicians preferred working with one person regarding the patient's entire hospital stay. The physician and the case manager designed "patient outcome plans" and "patient outcome timelines," which are analogous to the critical pathways.

When possible, the case manager contacts the physician and the patient prior to admission. At the time of admission, the case manager admits the patient to the unit and completes a thorough health history and initial assessment. Within the first 24 hours, the case manager reviews the patient outcome plan and patient outcome timeline. The plan is then reviewed with the nurse work group assigned to the actual delivery of care to that patient. The work group reviews the plan at the start of each shift, outlining specifics to be achieved during that shift. The case manager and the nurses group meet daily to evaluate outcomes and initiate any necessary modifications based on the patient's status. The case manager accompanies the physician during daily rounds to discuss progress and/or problems that need resolution.

Another example of leveled case management has been implemented at Hermann Hospital in Houston, Texas. This program is based on the principles of primary nursing with a career ladder consisting of six levels. Levels 1 and 2 are basic staff positions. Levels 3 through 6 involve responsibilities of a case manager. The nurses at levels 3 and 4 still maintain direct patient contact by directing care and monitoring compliance of the standards of practice, or the critical pathway. The case manager at level 5 is responsible for developing the standards of practice and ensuring cost-effective care and maximum utilization of resources. The nurse case managers at level 6 are clinical nurse specialists who are the liaisons among all members of the health care team. These case managers coordinate care with the other members of the team throughout the entire hospital stay, until discharge.[25]

Managerial or collaborative case management

Hussein Tahan attempted to further clarify the role of the nurse case manager by conducting a study in 1992 to develop a tool that could help identify and define the nurse case manager's role in the acute care setting. She categorized the role of the nurse case manager into three dimensions: clinical, managerial, and business or financial.[26]

The clinical dimension included assessing current health status, collecting information about past hospitalizations and medical history, establishing a nursing diagnosis, developing a care plan, and evaluating treatments.

The managerial role included planning care and length of stay related to DRG standards, developing a discharge plan, and facilitating communication among all members of the health care team. The nurse case manager acts as a supervisor to ensure the appropriate delivery of care, as a leader within the multidisciplinary group, and as a patient advocate to assess patient satisfaction. The nurse case manager in the managerial role is also responsible for conducting quality improvement activities.

The nurse case manager in the financial or business dimension works in collaboration with the other members of the health care team. The critical pathway is used as the tool to determine the most appropriate, time-efficient, and cost-effective treatment modality. The nurse case manager must have knowledge of the DRG structure to develop an appropriate plan of care and to evaluate financial outcomes. He or she works closely with the utilization review department in identifying problems and developing strategies to correct or prevent those problems.[27]

As the focus of case management continued to shift increasingly toward management, and away from clinical skills, facilities incorporated programs where the case manager not only was responsible for coordinating and monitoring patient care but also became increasingly responsible for issues related to insurance, reimbursement, and quality improvement.

The program developed at the 615-bed tertiary, nonprofit Tucson Medical Center in 1988 provides another example of the developing managerial role of the nurse case manager. Also referred to as the *Collaborative Case Management Model* and the *Arizona Model*, the main focus of this program is to standardize the use of patient resources during hospitalization for specific DRG case types.

The original proposal to incorporate case management into Tucson Medical Center indicates that the inability to control the process of care delivery was a major barrier to quality achievement. To overcome this barrier, 100 percent conformity of service had to be realized. To achieve this goal, "patient mix management" and "service volume management" strategies to control the process become more important than examining final outcomes. *Patient mix management* examines the number and type of patients admitted. Patient mix is also managed by channeling patients to alternative services, such as ambulatory centers or same day surgery sites. *Service volume management* maximizes the utilization of hospital resources. Resources include personnel as well as equipment, diagnostic tests, and procedures. A collaborative and multidisciplinary case management program seemed to be the most effective way of controlling the process, which would result in cost-effective, high-quality delivery of health care.

Using the New England Medical Center Hospital's model as a baseline, a multidisciplinary case management program was coordinated by nurses, using committees which included "hospital administrative personnel (human resources, medical staff administrator, finance department and case-mix coordinator); nursing personnel (administrative, management, all clinical areas, quality assurance, education and research); and other clinical staff (physical therapy, social services, dietary and rehabilitation)."[28] Subcommittees were formed at the unit-based level, where specific case type management programs were developed. The chair of the subcommittee was the nurse manager of that unit. From these committees and subcommittees, clinical practice patterns were reviewed and compiled to establish a standard of practice for each discipline.

As with NEMCH, a tool was developed to document the case management plan. However, since the New England case management plan includes nursing and medicine only, and the Tucson program is a collaborative effort, the case management plan was renamed the "Collaborative Case Management Plan" (CCMP). The CCMP detailed the specific standards of practice for a specific case type for each discipline involved in the patient's care. An abbreviated version of the CCMP, called the "CarePlan MAP," which is analogous to the generic critical pathway referred to above, becomes part of the permanent record.[29, 30]

One of the first case management programs to integrate a nursing theoretical background, Tucson Medical Center based its program on Dorothea Orem's model of selfcare. Orem's model is based on the belief that individuals will maintain a state of well being when they involve themselves in self-care activities.[31] Therefore, the CarePlan MAP also includes patient and family care activities. This focus assists the family in assuming a greater role as caretaker upon discharge. In today's cost-conscious environment, many home care needs are now the responsibility of the family. Inclusion of family educational needs while the patient is hospitalized facilitates a smooth and successful discharge and increased continuity of care.

Another modification to the NEMCH plan involved problem identification. In the NEMCH model, the identification of patient problems is at the core of the care process. The Tucson program, with a goal of promoting a strong nursing component, "identifies nursing's dependent, interdependent and independent components"[32] as the basis of care.

This system has multilevel nurse case managers. The hospital case management coordinator oversees the entire program. This position requires management and financial savvy. The coordinator is in direct communication with the group practice leaders, who coordinate the entire episode of care for a specific case type. The group practice leader works directly with the unit case managers to coordinate care across multiple nursing units. The unit-based nurse case manager provides direct care and coordinates care for those patients being case-managed on that unit. At each unit level there is also an associate case manager. Today, all case managers have a minimum of a baccalaureate degree. Nurses prepared at the diploma or associate degree level continue to provide direct patient care.

High-risk patients in each clinical area are assigned to a nurse case manager. Multidisciplinary committees are established, based on the specific DRG. For example, with a patient admitted for a total hip replacement, the team would include the physician, nurses from each unit involved with the patient's care, occupational and physical therapists, and the social worker. With a patient admitted for a laryngectomy, the team would include the physician, nurses, respiratory and speech therapists, and the social worker.

After 2 years, the results are impressive. Length of stay has been decreased by almost half in several DRG categories, length of stay in the more expensive intensive care units has dropped, and nursing satisfaction has increased significantly. It is reported that recruitment, hiring, and orienting a new nurse can cost from $8500 to $11,000 per nurse. At Tucson Medical Center, the turnover rate dropped from 29 percent to 5.3 percent during the pilot program, which has contributed to institutional cost savings.[33]

The collaborative case management program at Tucson Medical Center has been evolving to a "patient focused model," with quality as the major concern. Since 1993, CarePlan MAPs have been developed for all diagnoses, and remain the standard of care. The CCMP is no longer used. Nurses use flow sheets and focus charting, and traditional nursing notes having been eliminated.

In 1990, the University of Kentucky (UK) developed a program similar to the one at Tucson. However, instead of identifying patient concerns at a multidisciplinary advisory committee, the UK case managers are associated with physician groups. Problems, both clinical and financial, are identified within a specific specialty area through clinical experience and input from other health care providers, such as physicians, social workers, therapists, and dietitians. Suggestions are also received from administrators and finance personnel. Once the problems are identified, the component of the system responsible for the problem is discovered. When the problem lies within nursing, the case manager strategizes to resolve the problem and evaluates the clinical and financial outcomes. Collaboration becomes necessary in designing strategies when the problem lies outside the scope of nursing. In addition to consultation regarding the daily resolution of problems, the case manager meets with a case management advisory board on a quarterly basis for the purpose of identifying issues that cross specialty areas. [34]

In the UK program, the case manager is generally master's prepared, based on a study that indicated master's prepared nurses would be more likely to have the qualities of "collaboration/consultation skills, clinical expertise, and knowledge of evaluation."[35] "At the end of one year, data showed that case-managed patients went home 21.8 days earlier than comparable patients the previous year. In patient days, 872 were saved. For Medicaid patients alone, $82,731 was saved due to early discharge."[36]

THE FUTURE OF CASE MANAGEMENT IN ACUTE CARE

The changes in health care and the increasingly rapid formation of an integrated health care system have led to major shifts in the nursing profession in general, and case management in particular. The hospital is no longer the center of health care delivery but a component for continued movement through a growing system. Treatment is no longer begun at the outset of illness. Health care today is proactive in its approach, with the orientation of care being wellness and prevention, as opposed to cure. Health care today is quickly moving away from an acute illness model to one of chronic and complex disease management as well as primary prevention.

The case manager's role increasingly involves early problem identification, proactive coordination of care, decreasing hospital length of stay by coordinating transfer to a facility oriented toward caring for a lower acuity client, referring the patient to community support services, and continuing patient education to prevent recidivism or the occurrence of costly complications.

Managed care, capitated rates, shared risk, and formation of alliances have placed the case manager at a pivotal point. With an aim of increasing quality and decreasing cost, positive outcomes are impossible without a central person in charge of coordinating and communicating with the multiple providers involved in the delivery of care. Without the case manager, care will remain fragmented, continuous problem identification and timely resolution will not occur, and continuity of care will not be maintained across all units and boundaries.

Because of the added responsibilities given to the case manager and increased need for an expanding knowledge base, nurses prepared at the diploma and associate degree level will have fewer opportunities for employment. The baccalaureate and master's prepared nurses will find their niche increasingly in the field of case management.

As health care continues to become integrated, nurse case managers will find that they are "system case managers."[37] Acute care facilities are being forced to align themselves with networks of providers in order to remain viable. The case manager, at the center of this network, will be responsible for coordinated movement through the system.

As the central core of these networks and the person accountable for positive outcomes and continuous quality improvement (CQI), the case manager will need a fundamental understanding of systems theory. Systems theory is based on the importance of studying the whole as opposed to studying the parts. Being a theory of holism and synergism, it emphasizes the dynamic relationship between the individual and the environment. According to Kurt Lewin, a noted systems theorist, behavior is the result of the forces in the environment and the individual, working together. The environmental forces are psychobiological and are dynamic in nature. In Lewin's framework the individual does not simply respond to the environment but in fact chooses objects of interest and initiates action.[38]

To successfully coordinate movement through complex established networks, feedback, or the exchange of energy and information, will be an integral part of the case manager's role. The case manager must have a fundamental understanding of the hierarchical nature of systems and subsystems and of how one part of the system affects the operation of the other subsystems.

For the newly diagnosed, or catastrophically injured, the case manager in the acute care facility is often the lead person in the chain of providers. She or he is the one who will begin the orientation process. Whether the specific facility uses a primary nurse case management model, leveled care, or collaborative care will not be as significant as the skills of the nurse case manager at coordinating and facilitating care within a multileveled, multidisciplined environment.

Since the focus of health care delivery is now proactive, concurrent review is taking precedence over retrospective review. As a result, many of the responsibilities of the utilization review nurse will be assumed by the case manager. Discharge planning has become a component of the case management process and will therefore eliminate the need for many of the discharge planner's functions. To eliminate overlapping of role functions and to avoid duplication of services, departments are merging, and added responsibilities are being given to the nurse case manager. For example, St. Michael Hospital in Milwaukee, Wisconsin, merged its case management department with the utilization management and social work departments. At this time, social workers are involved only with patient and family counseling. There is a decreased focus on utilization review, with the majority of responsibilities performed by the nurse case manager.[39]

Tucson Medical Center's collaborative case management program is also evolving toward a unification of the utilization review department and the discharge planning department. Although this is a highly collaborative effort, many of the discharge functions are in the realm of the nurse case manager.

As the nursing profession gains accountability, credibility, and increased responsibility, the role of the nurse case manager will continue to expand and modify with the changing times.

COMMUNITY-BASED CASE MANAGEMENT

As the growth of case management programs in acute care facilities continued to expand, modify, and adapt to the ever-changing health care environment, it became evident that the most successful case management models would encompass managing care beyond the boundaries of the institution.

Carondelet St. Mary's Hospital and Health Center, in Tucson, Arizona, a 374-bed acute care facility, developed one of the first "beyond the walls" nurse case manager programs. This is also one of the few case management programs that has incorporated a nursing theory. Carondelet's program reflects Margaret Newman's theory of "health and expanding consciousness." Newman's theory is based on movement, space, and time—the three dimensions of consciousness. People's interactions with each other or their environment create patterns. Nursing can help patients identify those patterns and become aware of available choices. According to Newman, as making decisions becomes easier, the patient moves to a higher level.[40] Thus, the nurses at Carondelet assist the patient in identifying various patterns and then help in promoting positive decisions through awareness of choice. As the decision-making process becomes easier, the patient reaches a higher level of consciousness.

The hospital, connected with 19 nurse-managed health centers, has traditionally developed programs to enhance the nursing profession. Programs such as acuity billing for nurses, salaried status, and shared governance have been in place for many years. *Acuity billing* is an accounting method which incorporates consideration of how much skilled nursing is required based on the patient's needs. Nurses who have *salaried status* are paid a fixed annual wage regardless of the number of hours required to fulfill the job description (there is no overtime for extra work). *Shared governance* offers participative status to staff nurses in the management of the institution. Nurses have the power to implement changes in the work environment in areas that impact on patient care and in areas outside the discipline of nursing.

In its first attempt at designing a case management program that would include continuing care beyond discharge, Carondelet developed a decentralized home care program: The hospital nurse followed the patient after discharge and provided home care. Although this design decreased fragmentation of care, evaluation of the program indicated that hospital nurses were not experienced enough in home care to project outcomes within predetermined time frames, which was necessary for reimbursement.

By 1986, the nursing department developed a network of nursing services, referred to as the "nursing network." Review of the literature indicates that the nursing network is also called "the home-based case management model," and "the professional nursing network model." This integrated system crosses the boundaries between the hospital and the community. The nurses, who have at least BSN preparation, are accountable for the quality and cost-effectiveness of care as well as for accessibility to health care.[41] The nurse case manager, at the center of this network, is responsible for moving the patient through the continuum of health care. Through collaborative efforts with a multidisciplinary team, the case manager is responsible for assessing the patient, establishing a plan of care, coordinating services, providing referral sources, initiating interventions, and evaluating outcomes. The development of this network is based on three assumptions relative to the nursing profession. According to Etheredge and Lamb these assumptions are:[42]

1. Quality of patient services is directly related to professional accountability
2. Quality of patient services is directly related to continuity of care and a holistic approach to patient and family needs.
3. Quality of patient services is related to the educational preparation of the nurses prescribing care.

Through this network, people in the community have access to a wide range of services, including acute care, rehabilitation, home health care, long-term care, hospice, primary preventive and ambulatory services.[43, 44] The population served includes the acutely ill, chronically ill, terminally ill, and those at high risk. All of the 19 health care centers are nurse managed and operate within a professional nursing group. With the nurse case manager at the center of the network, referrals are made to the appropriate professional. Each system is comprised of a cardiac rehabilitation nurse, acute care nurse, home health nurse, community nurse educator, diabetes nurse educator, pulmonary rehabilitation nurse, infusion professional nurse, and hospice nurse. In addition, ambulatory nursing centers and geriatric nurse specialists within skilled nursing facilities are part of the network.

Referrals are received from the community, the hospital, and physicians. Most of the referrals come from the hospital and are based on complexity, acuity level, and high risk status. "High risk status is determined by a number of criteria including (1) age of the patient; (2) age of the family caregiver; (3) number and frequency of previous admissions; and (4) potential complications, based on the presence of multiple health and social problems."[45]

In-patients are identified as high risk for readmission, such as the elderly, those with chronic illnesses, and those with poor support systems. The case manager is responsible for coordinating, planning, and evaluating patient education and providing community resource referrals. He or she makes home visits after discharge to provide emotional support, assess environmental factors that might influence exacerbation of an illness, and reinforce teaching related to self-care. The case manager is also the liaison among all members of the health care team and the community, in the event of readmission.

In this system, the hospital-based nurse case manager works with clients in the acute and chronic care facilities and then in their home settings, spending approximately 30 percent of her or his time inside the hospital and 70 percent in the community.[46] Each case manager is responsible for approximately 40 patients, 10 in the acute care and 30 in the community. In addition, the nurse may have an additional 50 patients who are stable and require only monthly phone contact.[47]

When the referral is received, the nurse case manager meets with the patient to establish a rapport and collect information related to current and past medical, psychosocial, environmental, and spiritual issues. This information is used to identify problems, design a course of nursing treatment, and initiate a discharge plan. In the role of liaison and facilitator, the nurse case manager then meets with a multidisciplinary team to achieve successful outcomes based on the planned goals. As the nurse case manager follows the patient through the hospital, and back into the community, or into an extended care facility, he or she evaluates and revises goals as problems are encountered or resolved.[48, 49, 50]

"Nursing wellness centers," a component of the nursing network, are community-based clinics. Within these nurse-managed centers, nurse practitioners provide health screening, counseling, and health promotion services to the elderly population. Screenings for blood pressure, cholesterol, and blood sugar are offered. Educational workshops are coordinated, as well as exercise programs, nutritional counseling, and stress reduction programs. Clients are referred to physicians when appropriate. Outcome data showed decreased hospital length of stay, reduced levels of acuity at readmission, and increased use of community resources.[51]

In 1990, continued evolution of the nursing case management program led to the development of a "nursing HMO." Under a per capita Senior Plan contract, the nursing division at Carondelet is managing the health care needs of approximately 15,000 elderly and disabled clients. Upon admission to the acute care facility, one or more of six criteria must be met for assignment to a case manager. The criteria are (1) physiologically imbalanced; (2) emotionally challenged; (3) have no caregiver; (4) has a caregiver with a knowledge deficit; (5) only qualifies for home health for a time but needs private services, homemaker, and/or respite services; and (6) chooses to stay in own home or consistently utilizes the emergency room or the hospital for immediate health care needs.[52] Approximately 8 percent of the covered lives fit this profile.

The 19 community clinics are the focal point of the HMO, with a goal of assisting the client to achieve a healthier lifestyle. The key functions of the nurse practitioners are "health promotion, prevention, monitoring of illness, and referrals."[53] Referrals are received from physicians, case managers, or people in the community. Collaboration with community volunteers is a way of providing necessary care and maintaining cost-effectiveness. After the first 11 months, data indicated an average reduction of "one third the number of inpatient days. This translates into $300,000 for every 1000 enrollees."[54]

Following the success with senior citizens of this nursing HMO, Carondelet St. Mary's began developing a multidisciplinary team of providers, facilitated by nursing, for intensive nursing case management for a higher-risk population. The case manager's role when caring for the high-risk population is to identify their needs, help them to realize the consequences of continuing with their present lifestyle, and then to assist them to reach a readiness to accept and use the available community resources.[55]

Most patients who have been candidates for case management in the acute care setting have ongoing health care needs which can be dealt with by continued case management in alternate settings. Patients are discharged either home or to a setting for lower acuity needs. These settings include:

- Rehabilitation institute
- Subacute facility
- Community agencies or home care

Case managers assume a different role in each of the settings. Before discussing the role of the case manager in these settings, it is important to understand the purposes, similarities, and differences among the various health care facilities.

THE NURSE CASE MANAGER IN THE REHABILITATION INSTITUTION

A rehabilitation facility "treats neuromuscular impairment, disability and handicap and works to restore persons with physical disabilities to their highest possible levels of physical, psychological, social, vocational, and economic functioning."[56] Rehabilitation for the physically disabled emerged as an important aspect of health care during World War II, when Dr. Howard D. Rusk demonstrated that physical and psychological care was more effective than convalescence in rehabilitating the soldier to a level where he or she was able to return to duty.[57]

From centers that were developed primarily for the amputees and paraplegics returning from battle, rehabilitation has evolved into a process that enables the injured or catastrophically diagnosed to return to an independent lifestyle as productive human beings.

Many rehabilitation facilities today specialize in treating specific injuries or diagnoses, such as spinal cord injuries, amputations, burns, neuromuscular diseases, or traumatic brain injuries.

With the advent of advanced technology and the ability to design highly functional adaptive equipment, the rehabilitation process has allowed the severely disabled to return to a functional and productive lifestyle. Passage of the Americans with Disabilities Act in 1990 further helped the disabled population to assimilate into mainstream society. It is estimated that through rehabilitation 300,000 Americans return to work, saving Medicaid and other insurers $1 to 2 billion per year. An additional $700 million is generated in federal and state income taxes.[58]

When working with the catastrophically injured population, it is important to realize that the individual is referred to as "the client" and not "the patient," as in the acute care facility. Catastrophically injured people are not ill, they are injured. Two categories of catastrophic injury follow.

Spinal Cord Injury

Spinal cord injury (SCI) is defined as, "damage to the spinal cord and distortion of adjacent structures that occur in traumatic injury."[59] It is estimated that 250,000 people in this country have spinal cord injuries, with an average of 11,000 new injuries per year. Fifty-five percent of the spinal cord injured are paraplegic, and 44 percent are quadriplegic. Motor vehicle accidents account for 40 percent of SCIs, 25 percent are the result of violence, 21 percent come from falls, and 10 percent come from diving accidents. The remaining 4 percent are a result of work-related or sports-related accidents.

Sixty percent of all spinal cord injuries occur between the ages of 16 and 30, with the most frequent occurring at age 19. Seventy percent of spinal cord injury victims are male. Ninety percent of spinal-cord-injured individuals survive and live near-normal lifespans.

Initial hospitalization averages 100 days. The cost, including adaptive equipment and home modifications, averages $140,000.

Additional lifetime costs average $600,000 and reach as high as $1.35 million, depending on severity of injury and age of occurrence. In 1992, there were 10,000 reported spinal cord injuries nationwide. The lifetime costs associated with these injuries are projected to total $10 billion.[60]

Traumatic Brain Injury

"Traumatic Brain Injury (TBI) is an insult to the brain, not of degenerative or congenital nature but caused by an external physical force that may produce a diminished or altered state of consciousness, which results in an impairment of cognitive abilities or physical functioning."[61] Every 15 seconds somebody in the United States sustains a head injury. Approximately 373,000 people are hospitalized annually with traumatic brain injury. Of these, 99,000 will have permanent disabling conditions. Fifty percent of head injuries are the result of motor vehicle accidents. Falls are the second cause of head injuries and account for more than 20 percent. Over 50 percent of those with traumatic brain injury have been intoxicated at the time of the injury. Males aged 14 to 24 years are at the highest risk, followed by infants and the elderly.

The cost of traumatic brain injury is estimated at $48.3 billion annually. Hospitalization alone accounts for approximately $31.7 billion.[62]

Essentials for Admission

Patients who are transferred to a rehabilitation facility are usually evaluated for appropriateness of placement while still in acute care. The two essential criteria are potential for rehabilitation and the ability to partake in a minimum of 3 hours of aggressive therapy daily.

Because there are so many ways to treat head injuries, those sustaining traumatic brain injury are usually admitted into a specialized facility. Since the highest level of functioning achieved depends upon the degree of disability, many traumatic brain injury treatment centers provide day programs for outpatient treatment, residential programs for both temporary and permanent residents, community reentry programs, and independent living centers, where minimal supervision is needed.

Clients can spend many months in a rehabilitation facility. They must relearn how to function independently, learn how to use the multitude of adaptive equipment available, often be reeducated vocationally, and journey through Elizabeth Kubler-Ross' five stages of loss, to integrate their deficits into the reality of their futures.

The Rehabilitation Team

Rehabilitation facilities can employ up to 11 or more health care providers responsible for care. Rehabilitation is an interdisciplinary effort even, in certain facilities such as Craig Hospital in Englewood, Colorado, transdisciplinary. At Craig, many of the professional staff are cross-trained. For example, although the physical therapist's responsibility is to teach the client how to transfer, every team member must know the technique and be capable of performing it.[63] The health care providers found in the rehabilitation facility are usually as follows:

- *Physiatrist (attending physician, specialized in rehabilitation medicine)*: The physiatrist is the admitting physician, responsible for prescribing therapy, maintaining medical stability, and recommending a comprehensive treatment plan. The physiatrist often continues to treat the client as an outpatient and becomes the primary physician after discharge.
- *Neuropsychiatrist (the attending physician in a head injury rehabilitation facility)*: A neuropsychiatrist addresses the cognitive, as well as behavioral and psychological problems evident after a traumatic brain injury.
- *Psychologist and/or neuropsychologist*: The psychologist and/or neuropsychologist is responsible for the psychological well-

being and sexuality issues of both the patient and the family. These issues are usually treated with both individual and group therapy. These providers also deal with cognitive problems that may result from an injury, as well as pain management and stress management.

- *Nurses*: The nursing team is responsible for the daily skilled care needed, and the nurses reinforce techniques and strategies learned in therapy. They teach family members how to implement nursing care to prepare for discharge home.
- *Physical therapist*: The physical therapist is responsible for maximizing gross motor skills, teaching clients and family members techniques and strategies for care.
- *Occupational therapist*: The occupational therapist is responsible for maximizing fine-motor coordination and teaching independence in activities of daily living. He or she is also responsible for designing and recommending various adaptive equipment as needed. In a collaborative effort with the physical therapist, recommendations are made regarding appropriate home modifications. The occupational therapist also teaches family members techniques and strategies for care.
- *Speech therapist*: The speech therapist is responsible for communication skills, focusing on restoring verbal communication if possible. A variety of adaptive equipment may also be used to facilitate the client's communication.
- *Recreational therapist*: The recreational therapist assists the client to function in society by integrating the skills learned in physical and occupational therapy. Therapeutic recreation involves taking the client into the community to learn socialization and living skills from the level of a wheelchair.
- *Vocational counselor*: The vocational counselor assists the patient in developing and attaining vocational goals.
- *Social worker*: The social worker works in conjunction with the case manager to coordinate care. She or he assists in procurement of local, state, or federal funding and refers the family and client to community support systems or programs.

- *Family member or significant other*: The family member(s) or significant other must learn to accept major life changes. Goals may need redefining. Economics and future planning may need restructuring. The family members must also be educated about the specific illness or injury and learn strategies and techniques of caregiving.
- *Other professionals*: In many institutions additional professionals include respiratory therapists, nutritionists, and aquatic therapists. Full-time respiratory care professionals are necessary when the facility cares for the client who is ventilator-dependent.
- *The case manager*: The case manager is at the hub of these multiple health care providers. The role of the case manager will be discussed in more depth later in this chapter.

Planning Treatment

Treatment in rehabilitation is geared toward maximizing abilities and achieving the highest level of functioning within existing limitations. During the rehab process, issues needing to be addressed include maintenance of skin integrity, independence in activities of daily living, sexuality, vocational issues, psychological acceptance, and major changes in life planning. Since the average length of stay can range from several weeks to several months, health care providers have the benefit of time to establish an appropriate plan.

Many rehabilitation facilities have begun to adopt critical pathways as their guide to standardized treatment. Critical pathways are usually developed by the interdisciplinary team as a collaborative effort. However, due to the many uncontrollable variances and multiple levels of injury clients sustain, incorporating critical pathways into the rehabilitation process remains very difficult.[64] Research into effective standards of practice and evaluating outcomes continues. Whichever method of multidisciplinary and collaborative care plans is used, they all outline short-term and long-term goals. Each goal is measured along timelines of days, weeks, or months, depending upon the specific goal. Some long-term goals may be for a year or more, such as vocational and career goals or reaching total independence in all activities of daily living.

In most rehabilitation facilities, physician-led team meetings are held monthly. All disciplines involved in the client's care attend, and each provider gives a verbal overview of the progress, goals, and obstacles experienced during the previous month. Many times the client is present through part of or all the meeting. Usually the external case manager is also present to assess the current status, goals, and discharge time frames. Continued verification of payment or limits to coverage are discussed. After each provider gives a verbal update, the members strategize to resolve variances, make recommendations for treatments, and set new goals for the next 4-week period. Since strong communication between disciplines is important for successful rehabilitation, in addition to these monthly meetings, many of the providers may meet or communicate on a daily or weekly basis.

The Role of the Nurse Case Manager

The role of the nurse case manager in the rehabilitation facility differs somewhat from that of the case manager in the acute care setting. In the acute care facility the major focus is to manage disease. In rehabilitation the focus is to manage life. Although the underlying process of case management remains similar in both the acute care facility and the rehabilitation institution, the dominant population in rehabilitation is the young adult who is well but injured. The patient within the acute care facility is generally older, with an acute episode of an illness. In addition, the length of time as an inpatient is much longer in the rehabilitation facility, which allows for more in-depth case management. Whereas the goal of the case management process in the acute care facility is to achieve a higher level of wellness, the goal of the case management process in the rehabilitation facility is to achieve a higher level of functioning and independence.

The case manager is responsible for maintaining continuity of care, coordinating movement through the rehabilitation process, and ensuring a smooth transition at discharge. The case manager is the liaison among the members of the team involved in the client's care. He or she collaborates directly with the external or insurance-based, case manager, to verify payment and to relay the specific services and/or equipment needs at discharge, so that a smooth transition from facility to facility or facility to home can occur. The case manager's responsibilities also include referring to community support services and assisting significant others with the ramifications of family dynamics. The case manager in the rehab facility is the person that the family and the patient turn to for answers.

Coordination of home care for the catastrophically injured is a major and expensive undertaking. Frequently home modifications are necessary to allow for accessibility for the injured person. Adaptive equipment and devices are required for independent living. Many times the patient will require the services of a home health aide or more highly skilled home care providers. In today's health care environment, payment for services and/or equipment is a major concern. Many third-party payers do not cover much of the required care, or they place a cap on their policies so that coverage may be used up prior to the client's discharge home. Most families are unable to afford the multitude of services necessary to ensure a high level of independent living. State funding, as well as both Medicare and Medicaid, do not cover many of the necessities required. Although in past years the state departments of vocational rehabilitation would often provide necessary equipment and services for the purpose of career reeducation and independent living, currently much of the necessary funding is unavailable due to budget cuts.

Historically, nurses have been averse to discussing the financial aspects of health care with clients. In today's cost-conscious and cost-effective health care environment, the financial aspect cannot be pushed aside. The cost of health care has become an integral part of the planning process. An intricate and detailed plan of care, without provision for payment, is useless. The case manager's ability to coordinate appropriate care depends upon the creative use of limited funds and knowledge of community resources, as well as legal, insurance, and vocational issues.

The role of the case manager in the rehabilitation facility can be divided into five basic functions: (1) assessing, (2) planning, (3) coordinating, (4) implementing, and (5) evaluating. These functions will be discussed in depth in Chapter 7.

THE NURSE CASE MANAGER IN THE SUBACUTE FACILITY

The Joint Commission for the Accreditation of Health Organizations (JCAHO) defines subacute as

> [C]omprehensive inpatient care designed for someone who has had an acute illness, injury, or exacerbation of a disease process. It is goal-oriented treatment rendered immediately after, or instead of, acute hospitalization to treat one or more specific active complex medical conditions or to administer one or more technically complex treatments, in the context of a person's underlying long term conditions and overall situation. Generally, the individual's condition is such that the care does not depend heavily on high technology monitoring or complex diagnostic procedures. It requires the coordinate services of an interdisciplinary team including physicians, nurses, and other relevant professional disciplines, who are trained and knowledgeable to assess and manage these specific conditions and perform the necessary procedures. It is given as part of a specifically defined program, regardless of the site.
>
> Subacute care is generally more intensive than traditional nursing facility care and less than acute care. It requires frequent (daily to weekly) recurrent patient assessment and review of the clinical course and treatment plan for a limited (several days to several months) time period, until a condition is stabilized or predetermined treatment course is completed.[65]

In essence, a *subacute facility* can be defined as the facility that bridges the gap between acute care and home.[66]

Development of Subacute Care

It is reported that in any acute care hospital with more than 250 beds, "3 percent of all admissions account for about 20 percent of all patient days."[67] It is also estimated that "16 percent of individuals receiving care for chronic conditions require 41 percent of the total dollar expenditure."[68]

Subacute facilities proliferated as an outgrowth of the health care reform of the 1990s. Alternative facilities were needed to fill the gap for those patients who would benefit from rehab but did not fit the criteria for the comprehensive rehabilitation facilities, were not appropriate for nursing home placement, and were too medically unstable to return home. Until the advent of the concept of sub-acute care, these people remained in the more expensive acute care hospital beds.

As the health care system continues to shift toward managed care, where the philosophy is one of shared risk and reduction of delivery costs, there has been an emergence of alternative and cost-effective care. The subacute industry offers skilled nursing or re-habilitation strategies to deliver an appropriate level of care at a reduced cost to accommodate patients who would otherwise have to remain in an acute care setting.

The proliferation of subacute units found within acute care institu-tions has been motivated by the need to increase the number of occu-pied beds and remain solvent. Fierce competition among hospitals, decreased reimbursement, and shortened length of stay have fueled the need to develop alternative models of care as a means of survival. Many skilled nursing facilities have developed subacute programs that offer a higher level of care and bring in increased reimburse-ment from insurance carriers. There is also the benefit of attracting a broader scope of the patient population which can be served.

The concept of subacute care has not been in existence long enough to compile outcome measures and statistics. The process of data collection continues, with experts in the field generally optimistic that the final figures will indicate that using subacute as alternative treatment will result in large dollar savings. Critics of subacute, however, have maintained that the industry tends to be "proprietary driven" and will lead to overuse of services to increase profits.[69]

Characteristics of Subacute Care

Most of the subacute facilities have developed through Medicare certified nursing homes, Medicare certified long-term beds in acute care hospitals, and long-term hospitals that admit patients requiring a length of stay over 25 days. Although many admissions to the subacute are patients transferred from acute rehab, an equal number are transferred directly from acute care hospitalization. Patients are also admitted directly from home or from a nursing facility.

Many payers have differentiated between subacute rehab and subacute medical, for clarity of cost comparison. The primary population served in subacute rehab include the elderly who need to build endurance, individuals having reached a plateau in acute rehab, and others who are not capable of participating in the aggressive therapy programs in the acute rehabilitation facility. Individuals most commonly found in subacute rehab are catastrophically injured (including spinal cord injuries, traumatic brain injuries, or stroke) or require short-term rehab for orthopedic problems (hip or knee replacement). The general criterion for admission is an inability to tolerate 3 hours of therapy per day. In subacute rehab, individuals work within their own endurance levels.

Admissions for subacute medical are frequently based on treatment needs, such as IV therapy, chemotherapy, wound care, or ventilator management. Patients who benefit from subacute medical include those who have been diagnosed with HIV or AIDS-related diseases who require a higher level of care than can be provided at home for certain cancers or who have disease-related problems such as severe wound care needs.[70]

It is projected that as subacute becomes entrenched in the health care system, many traditional acute care patients, such as those undergoing open heart surgery or organ transplantation, will spend much of their recuperative period in subacute facilities. Some experts in the field are currently developing a model to incorporate subacute prior to the acute care stay for the purpose of strengthening, educating, and orienting. As an example, the person undergoing knee replacement would be admitted to a subacute facility several days prior to the surgery. Strengthening and conditioning exercises, along with education, will likely decrease the time needed for the postoperative rehab process.[71]

As with the rehabilitation facilities, use of critical pathways is often difficult due to the presence of comorbidities and uncontrollable variances. However, since the critical pathways remain an application of the CQI principles and document established standards of care, most subacute facilities continue their efforts to integrate the critical pathways into their treatment plans. The goal of the subacute critical pathway is to improve quality by identifying complications of a chronic condition, or exacerbation, at an earlier date than traditionally.[72]

Role of the Case Manager

The case manager in the subacute facility has many of the same goals as the case manager in the rehab facility. The differences, however, revolve around the patient population—which is more heterogeneous than in the acute rehabilitation facility and with respect to level of independence projected and time frames for discharge. The average length of stay in a subacute facility is 2 to 3 weeks.

The role of the case manager in the subacute facility is vital. Since the treatment of subacute patients is individualized to their specific endurance level, problem identification and strategizing to resolve variances remain difficult. The case manager, as the person accountable for positive outcomes, must create an environment of collaborative and interdisciplinary communication on a continuous basis to maximize the outcomes of resources used, prevent increased length of stay, and coordinate timely implementation of care.

Subacute facilities conduct team meetings comparable to those in acute rehab. The case manager is at the hub of the multidisciplinary providers, coordinating care among and between all providers. The discharge needs discussed at these meetings usually involve additional assistance in the home. Since family members have been assuming a larger share of the home care responsibilities, a key to successful case management is in arranging support services for the home.[73]

The basic five functions outlined under the role of case manager in the acute rehab facility also apply to the case manager in the subacute facility.

THE NURSE CASE MANAGER AND HOME CARE

Most patients admitted to acute care are discharged directly to home. However, many need the coordination of home care services, on either a temporary or permanent basis. The case manager plays a vital and ongoing role in the coordination and cost containment of home care services.

Types of Home Care Agencies

There are two basic financial structures of home care agencies. There are *nonprofit agencies*, which fall under the visiting nurses associations (VNAs), and there are *proprietary for-profit agencies*. Until recently, hospital personnel would generally refer clients with home care needs to the VNA. However, as a government controlled agency, the VNA can only do skilled nursing visits. As hospital length of stay has become shorter, the acuity level of patients returning home has increased. The outcome has been a growing demand for home care service ranging from support in ADL (activities of daily living) to highly technical skilled nursing care. To meet the range of home care needs, there has been growth in the proprietary nursing agency sector. To maintain their place in the health care arena, the VNAs have recently begun to develop proprietary components. Hospitals also have entered the competitive market by developing their own proprietary home care departments. Today, both proprietary and nonprofit home care agencies are found within the community and within many acute care facilities.

In the early to mid-1990s, when home care was seen as a more cost-effective alternative to hospitalization, home care agencies proliferated. Competition led to the need for the individual agencies to cover larger geographic areas. The changing focus of health care and demographics led to the formation of fewer but larger "total care" agencies, many of which formed consortia that now can provide services to entire regions. Many of these larger organizations have contracted with providers of ancillary services to form preferred provider organizations (PPOs). With the advent of PPOs, and increasing need for cost containment, many proprietary agencies have contracted with various hospitals and are now in stronger competition with the nonprofit agencies. As of December 1994, there were a total of 13,343 home care agencies throughout the United States. That is a growth of 16 percent over 1993.[74]

Characteristics of Home Care

With the explosive growth of managed care and continued efforts to decrease hospital length of stay, more patients are being discharged home who have continued need for skilled care. Many times homes are transformed into "minihospitals," and home care agencies are proliferating to fill this niche. Today, most home care agencies are equipped to provide appropriate care to the patient who is still acutely ill or who needs high-tech equipment and nurses with experience in critical care.

As a result of corporate growth, home care agencies today have several layers of management. Level 1 is the home care supervisor, the person directly responsible for overseeing every aspect of care. (For the purpose of this book, discussion of the role of the nurse case manager in home care will be limited to the nursing supervisor who is the person directly involved with coordinating patient care.)

Prior to discharge from the acute care, rehabilitation, or subacute setting, the home care supervisor, or case manager, performs an initial patient evaluation in the facility. A complete health history is taken, which includes past medical history, admitting diagnosis, and current treatment plan. An important part of the data collection is an assessment of possible problems at home that may interfere with the success of a home care plan. The patient's knowledge base, motivation level, compliance, and support system greatly affect the positive outcomes of home care.

The Role of the Case Manager

The case manager works in a joint effort with the facility case manager to coordinate a smooth discharge home and maintain continuity of care. Since the in-house case manager has been working collaboratively with the multidisciplinary providers in the specific setting, she or he is cognizant of discharge needs regarding durable medical equipment (DME), supplies, and/or continued need for ancillary services such as physical, occupational, speech, or respiratory therapy. The level and frequency of nursing care depend upon the needs of the patient and the knowledge base and support of the family structure.

Based on the data collection, a complete plan of care is outlined. Critical pathways are infrequently used in proprietary home care because of the large number of uncontrollable variables. As an example, two patients are discharged home who are ventilator-dependent. They are both alert and oriented. Patient A has a knowledgeable, supportive family structure, anxious to assist in the responsibilities of care; patient A is married, and his wife is not employed outside the home. The house is clean, well kept, and organized. Patient A might be discharged to home with 12 hours/day of RN care. The RN is able to teach the family how to perform suctioning, tracheostomy care, and ventilator maintenance. They can be taught how to ambu the patient in the event of a ventilator failure and given instructions for emergency treatment. In this case, after several weeks, this patient may need only weekly or biweekly skilled nursing visits.

Patient B is also discharged to home with 12 hours/day of RN care. Patient B is married; however, his wife is employed full-time and spends an additional 2 hours per day commuting. In addition, the patient's extended family is not supportive and is unwilling to take on any of the skilled care needs. The family has a large dog that is allowed the "run of the house" and was observed sniffing the suction and tracheostomy care supplies. Patient B will require skilled nursing needs for a much longer time than patient A to prevent rehospitalization. The goal in caring for patient A is the reduction of the level and frequency of nursing care. The goal for patient B is avoidance of repeat hospitalization. Both plans might have positive outcomes; however, a critical pathway for ventilator-dependent home care would have limitations in both scenarios.

Nonprofit home care agencies have begun to develop critical pathways based on the limited visits allowed through Medicare reimbursement. For example, a VNA nurse may be assigned to a patient newly diagnosed with chronic obstructive pulmonary disease (COPD) to teach the use of an inhaler and nebulizer. Medicare guidelines dictate the maximum allowed visits. The critical pathway would be developed within these time frames.

After all the needs are assessed and the complete plan of care is outlined, the insurance carrier is contacted by the home care case manager to assess the particular policy benefits. Once approval is received from the payer, the case manager coordinates all additional care within the PPO and continues to work collaboratively with the other providers during the time that services are needed.

Many skilled needs in the home can be performed by a licensed practical nurse (LPN). Often the physician is unaware of the differences in licensure and orders RN services. It is the role of the nurse case manager to review the necessary skill level and place the appropriate nurse in the home in collaboration with the physician. The nurse case manager's professional responsibility is to provide care in the most cost-effective manner possible, without compromising quality.

The goal of the nurse case manager in home care is to use allocated resources in the most cost-effective manner in an ever-changing environment. An example would be a policy limit on supplies, such as suction catheters. In such an event, the home care nurse would use sterilization techniques in order to reuse the catheters. In this manner, the patient can receive appropriate treatment, reduce out-of-pocket costs, and remain within the scope of the policy benefit package.

The nurse case manager is also responsible for ensuring complete home care staffing, speaking with the patient on a weekly basis to assess status and discussing any problems regarding home care services. The case manager visits the patient on a monthly basis and evaluates every staff member on a monthly basis. Problem identification is a continual process, with resolution of the problem a collaborative effort among the nursing and ancillary staff, the family, the patient, and the physician.

Since most policy benefits have a limit on services and equipment and/or supply needs, the role of the nurse case manager in home care is to assist with coordinating appropriate care beyond the scope of third-party payer benefits. The home care nurse must be knowledgeable regarding local, state, and federal resources and must have complete knowledge of Medicare and Medicaid eligibility requirements, available waivers, and other avenues to research to maintain appropriate and high-quality care.

One issue that the home care case manager must deal with— which other case managers do not—is that of abandonment. Once a case is accepted, the nursing agency cannot just "walk away," regardless of the reason. If an agency wants to discontinue care, the patient and the patient's attorney (if one exists) must receive written notice, 72 hours in advance. In addition, the family and attorney must be given alternative agencies to call, or alternative methods of care, such as information about inpatient facilities.

Chapter Highlights

* Internal case management developed within the acute care setting as a means of coordinating cost-effective care without compromising quality.

* Institutions have focused on developing models to guide case management practice. The models are referred to by many terms including *critical pathway*, *clinical pathway*, *CareMap*, and *MAP*. In essence, all models strive to provide a system for identifying variances that may delay positive outcomes. The pathways also are used for standardizing treatment.
* The role of the internal nurse case manager is to focus on strategies to predict and resolve these variances.
* Clients receive care across a continuum of settings. The case manager participates in determining the most appropriate setting for care. The usual goal is to select the least expensive facility that can promote satisfactory client outcomes.
* Successful case management is accomplished by "passing the torch" from one level of care to another, through collaborative and multidisciplinary efforts.

References

1. Thomas, C. (1993). *Tabors cyclopedic medical dictionary.* (17th ed.) Philadelphia, PA: FA Davis, p. 914.
2. Insurance Information Institute. (1995). *The fact book 1996: Property/casualty insurance facts.* New York. pp. 107–108.
3. Zander, K. (1988, May). Nursing case management: Strategic management of cost and quality outcomes. *Journal of Nursing Administration.* 18(5), 23.
4. Clark, M. (1996). *Nursing in the community.* (2d ed.) San Diego, CA: Appleton & Lange. p. 241
5. Zander, Nursing case management, p. 28.
6. Zander, K. (1985, Mar.). Second generation primary nursing a new agenda. *The Journal of Nursing Administration.* 15(3), 18.
7. Zander, K., Etheredge, M., & Bower, K. (1987). *Nursing case management: blueprints for transformation.* Waban, MA: Winslow. p. 12.
8. Zander, K. (1994, fall). Case management series part II: Identifying patient populations for case management. *The New Definition,* 9(4), 1.
9. Zander, Nursing case management, p. 23.
10. Cohen, E. & Cesta, T. (1993). *Nursing case management from concept to evaluation.* St. Louis: Mosby. p. 117.

11. Boling, J. (1992, July, Aug., Sept.). An American integrated health system? Where are we now? *The Case Manager*. 3(3), 57.

12. Zander, K. (1995, winter). Case management series part III: Case manager role dimensions. *The New Definition*, 10(1), back cover.

13. Boling, American integrated health system, p. 57.

14. Bower, K. (1992). *Case management by nurses*. Washington DC: American Nurses. p. 43.

15. Zander, Nursing case management, p. 23.

16. Ibid, p. 24.

17. Zander, Case manager role dimensions, p. 1.

18. Zander, K. (1991, Jan.). Case management in acute care: making the connections. *The Case Manager*. 2(1), 40.

19. Sinnen, M., & Schifalacqua, M. (1991, Mar.). Coordinated care in a community hospital. *Nursing Management*. 22(3), 40.

20. Ibid.

21. McKenzie, C., Torkelson, N., & Holt, M. (1989, Oct.). Care and cost: nursing case management improves both. *Nursing Management*. (20)10, 30.

22. Rotkovitch, R., & Smith, C. (1987, Nov.). ICON I—the future model. ICON II—the transition model. *Nursing Management*, 18(11).

23. Loveridge, C., Cummings, S., & O'Malley, J. (1988, Oct.). Developing case management in a primary nursing system. *The Journal of Nursing Administration*. 18(10), 38.

24. Ibid., p. 37.

25. Cavouras, C., Walts, L., Taylor, A., & Bordelon, P. (1990). Alternative delivery system: Primary case management. *Patient care delivery models*. Rockville, MD, Aspen Publishing. pp. 275–284.

26. Tahan, H. (1993, Oct.). The nurse case manager in acute care settings. *The Journal of Nursing Administration*. 23(10), 53.

27. Tahan, Acute care settings, pp. 53–61.

28. Guadalupe, O., Del Togno-Armanasco, V., Erickson, J., & Harter, S. (1989, Dec.). Case management—a bottom-line care delivery model part II: Adaptation of the model. *The Journal of Nursing Administration*. 19(12), 12–13.

29. Del Togno-Armanasco, V., Hopkin, L., & Harter, S. (1993). *Collaborative nursing case management: a handbook for development and implementation*. New York: Springer, p. 952.

30. Guadalupe, Del Togno-Armanasco, Erickson & Harter, Bottom-line care delivery model, pp. 14–15.

31. Clark, *Nursing in the community*, p. 952.

32. Guadalupe, Del Togno-Armanasco, Erickson, & Harter, Bottom-line care delivery model, p. 14.

33. Del Togno-Armanasco, V., Hopkin, L., & Harter, S. (1993). *Collaborative nursing case management: a handbook for development and implementation*. New York: Springer. p. 148.

34. Brockopp, D., Porter, M., Kinnaird, S., & Silberman, S. (1992, Sept.). Fiscal and clinical evaluation of patient care: a case management model for the future. *Journal of Nursing Administration*. 22(9), 24.

35. Ibid., p. 23.

36. Ibid., p. 27.

37. Beckley, N. (1995, Fall). Case management and integrated delivery. *Case Review*. 1(2), 25.

38. Haber, J., Leach, A, Schudy, S. & Sideleau, B. (1978). *Comprehensive psychiatric nursing*. New York: McGraw-Hill. p. 53.

39. Sinnen, M. Telephone conference, Nov. 29, 1995.

40. Etheredge, P. (1991, July). A nursing HMO: Carondelt St. Mary's experience. *Nursing Management*. 22(7), 23.

41. Etheredge, P., & Lamb, G. (1989, Mar.). Professional nursing case management improves quality, access and costs. *Nursing Management*. 20(3), 30.

42. Ibid.

43. Cohen & Cesta, *Concept to evaluation*, p. 44.

44. Bower, *Case management by nurses*, p. 30.

45. Etheredge & Lamb, Quality, access and costs, p. 31.

46. Bower, *Case management by nurses*, p. 29.

47. Etheredge, A nursing HMO, p. 30.

48. Lamb, G. (1992, Dec.). Conceptual and methodological issues in nurse case mangement research. *Advances in Nursing Science*. 15(2), 21.

49. Bower, *Case management by nurses*. pp. 29–33.

50. Etheredge, A nursing HMO, pp. 22–29.

51. Cohen & Cesta, *Concept to evaluation*, p. 44.

52. Etheredge, A nursing HMO: Carondelt St. Mary's experience. *Nursing Management*. 22(7), 24.

53. Ibid., p. 25.

54. Ibid., p. 26.

55. Smith, I. (1995, Fall). New models for case management. *Case Review*. 1(2), 17–22.

56. *The 1995 Grolier multimedia encyclopedia*. (1995). ISBN 07172-3981-0. [CD-ROM]

57. Ibid.
58. Huey, F. (1995, Sept. 5). Humpty Dumpty: good egg for rehab? *Nursing Spectrum.* 7A(18), 3.
59. Phipps, W., Long, B, & Woods, N. (1979). *Medical-surgical nursing.* St. Louis, MO: Mosby. p. 718.
60. American Paralysis Association (1995). Untitled fact sheet. The University of Alabama National Spinal Cord Injury Statistical Center, The Dana Alliance for Brain Initiatives and Paralyzed Veterans of America.
61. Brain Injury Association, Inc. (1995). Fax communication. Edison, NJ
62. Brain Injury Association, Inc. (1995). Fax communication. Edison, NJ
63. Daus, C. (1995, Fall). Seamless rehab. *Case Review,* 1(2), 64.
64. Ibid., p. 67.
65. The Joint Commission on Accreditation of Health care Organizations. (fax transmission Jan. 16, 1996). Accreditation Protocol for Subacute Programs.
66. Lee, R. (1995, Fall). Maximizing the continuum. *Case Review.* 1(2), 74.
67. Ibid.
68. Kelly, M. (1994, Fall). The intrinsic value of subacute services. *Journal of Subacute Care.* 1(3), 17.
69. Lee, Maximizing the continuum, p. 75.
70. Ibid., p. 74.
71. Ibid., p. 75.
72. Musfeldt, C., & Smith, J. (1994, Fall). Subacute care critical pathways: the road to cost-effective care and quality outcomes. *Journal of Subacute Care.* 1(3), 21–22.
73. Worsowicz, G., Stark-Reed, A., & Dinnerman, K. (1995, June). Subacute care—finding the appropriate level of care. *NJ Rehab.* pp. 15–17.
74. Newsbytes. (1995, Oct./Nov./Dec.). Sixteen percent more home health agencies. *The Case Manager.* 6(5), 6.

Role of 6
the External
Case Manager

In 1970, Americans spent $74 billion for health care, and estimates of the cost of health care in the year 2000 come to $1616 billion.[1] The escalating cost of health care has been the driving force behind the proliferation of all methods of case management. External case management developed parallel to, but separately from, case management in the acute care facility.

External case management—that is, any case management done by someone not employed by a health care facility or network (acute care hospital, rehabilitation institute, or subacute facility)— emerged in the 1970s as an effective means of controlling the costs of catastrophic illnesses and injuries. Until the mid-1990s, external case management evolved and grew as the health care industry grew. Traditional health insurance companies hired case managers to oversee their high dollar claims. Workers' compensation insurance carriers began using case managers not only to reduce the cost of medical treatment but also to achieve a timely return to work. Independent case management companies proliferated and marketed their services to the insurance industry and to large self-insured corporations.

External case managers may work directly for insurance carriers or managed care organizations (MCOs). Alternatively, external case managers can represent insurance carriers while employed by private case management companies. External case managers may also be in private practice, working directly for a client in need of such service.

Upon completion of this chapter you will be able to answer the following questions:

1. What are the pros and cons of telephonic case management?
2. How does the external case manager use the process of negotiation?
3. How does the external case manager develop and apply the skills of marketing, networking, and investigating?
4. In what ways does the role of the case manager vary according to the employment setting?
5. How is the role of the external case manager evolving in the independent and private practice arenas?

When working with clients injured in work-related accidents, external case managers are often referred to as "rehab nurses" or "rehab nurse/case managers." This term is also used for the nurse case manager working with the client diagnosed with spinal cord injury or traumatic brain injury. Many independent case management companies have two case management departments. The medical case management (MCM) department employs nurses who work with clients filing claims through their health insurance. The rehab department hires nurses working with clients filing workers' compensation or motor vehicle claims.

MANAGED CARE VERSUS MANAGED COMPETITION

In 1994, when health reform became a national issue, the growth of managed care, the formation of preferred provider organizations (PPOs), the formation of physician networks and alliances, and capitated rates had a tremendous impact on the role of the external case manager. Case management is not synonymous with managed care or managed competition. Managed care is a system of programs directed toward cost containment. Within the scope of managed care are health maintenance organizations (HMOs), preferred provider organizations (PPOs), physician-hospital organizations (PHOs) and point of service plans (POSs). (See Chapter 3.)

Managed competition, a phrase coined in 1970 by Alain Enthoven, referred to the mechanism that managed care programs used to obtain and maintain business. In the late 1970s sponsors or brokers examined available health plans, negotiated the costs, and offered their clients the plans that best suited their needs. Today these brokers are called health insurance purchasing cooperatives (HIPCs).[2]

Managed competition has evolved over four stages:

1. The "unstructured stage" saw the independent growth of hospitals and physicians without an organized purchasing system.
2. The "loose framework stage" saw the growth of managed care and the formation of provider networks.
3. The "consolidation stage" evolved as a few large purchasers of health care emerged. During this stage private practices began to disappear as systems of care grew.
4. The "managed competition" stage has begun to see physicians, hospitals, and insurance carriers unite and form integrated networks to manage the patient population.[3]

The speed of change in the health care arena has resulted in the rapid emergence of an integrated delivery system. What took 20 years to emerge in the west has evolved within months in the midwestern and eastern states.

The development of capitated rates, shared risk, and increased consolidation has resulted in a shift in the role of the nurse case manager. Case management is no longer viewed as a panacea only for catastrophic injuries and illnesses, it is also known as a method of reducing the cost of health care to a wide variety of clients through appropriate anticipatory planning, coordination, and implementation of care. As *preventive care* became the buzzword throughout the health care community in general, it became a catalyst for the continuing evolution of case management.

In summary, managed care is a system, and managed competition is a service. Case management, a process of delivering care, is a component of managed care and managed competition.[4] This chapter will explore both the traditional and emerging roles of the external nurse case manager in various settings.

DEFINITION OF TERMS

Utilization Review

Utilization review (UR) is a system which can help reduce unnecessary hospital admissions and control the length of stay for inpatients through evaluations and discharge planning.[5] Both hospitals and insurance companies employ UR nurses. Some case management firms have established independent utilization review departments. The goal of UR is appropriate and cost-effective utilization of services.

Utilization review is implemented in three ways: *Prospective review*, also called *precertification* or *preadmission*, determines medical appropriateness for admission to an acute care facility, rehabilitation institute, subacute facility, or same-day surgery center. The physician, or other provider of services, contacts the UR nurse with the following information: diagnosis, explanation of the medical necessity of the proposed treatment, and projected length of stay for the patient. If appropriate the UR nurse approves the admission. If the UR nurse denies the admission or service, the provider will need to offer additional data to establish medical necessity. In many instances, as stated in policy benefit packages, if precertification has not been received, the insurance carrier may not reimburse the full fee to the provider of services.

Concurrent review is performed throughout the duration of the event. The utilization review nurse contacts the provider of services at specific times. If the patient is in the intensive care unit, the UR nurse may contact the physician every day or two. If the patient is in a rehabilitation facility, reassessment would not be as frequent.

Retrospective review is performed following the completion of provided services or after discharge from a facility. A retrospective review is used to audit hospital bills to ensure overcharging has not occurred or to review appropriateness of the DRG (diagnosis-related group) that was assigned at the time of patient discharge. If the data obtained by retrospective review do not support the DRG, the UR nurse will renegotiate the DRG assigned.

Utilization Management

Utilization management (UM) is a relatively new term used to describe the joined processes of utilization review and case management. When it became apparent that utilization review alone was not generating the cost savings anticipated, utilization review was combined with case management in an attempt to manage high-dollar claims in a more cost-effective manner.

Through utilization management, a "red flag" system identifies selected claims for referral to case management services. Applying predetermined selection criteria, the UM nurse reviews all patient admissions and separates out those people who are likely to generate expensive claims. For example, a UM nurse who precertifies hospitalization for a client with a spinal cord injury would immediately refer the client for case management services. A UM nurse working directly for the insurance carrier assumes the role of the nurse case manager. If an independent UR/UM firm is used by the carrier, the reviewer would refer the claim to a nurse case manager working within that company. Utilization management nurses perform the role of nurse case manager telephonically, on-site, or in combination.

METHODS OF EXTERNAL CASE MANAGEMENT

Telephonic Case Management

Telephonic case management utilizes only the telephone for data collection and coordination of care (there is no direct, face-to-face client contact). Fax machines and computers allow for immediate transmission of records for review (see Chapter 11 for cautions for fax use.)

The two main advantages of telephonic case management are: (1) it is the least costly method for insurance carriers, and (2) the nurse case manager can handle cases over a broad geographic area (even nationwide). Among the several disadvantages to using the telephone as the sole means of data collection are:

1. The telephone is a limited medium for communication. Only verbal messages can be transmitted. Good communication for responsible data collection involves substantially more than "just words."

2. It is difficult to establish good rapport telephonically. Clients may feel anxious and inhibited about discussing topics that for them are of a delicate nature. Confidentiality issues may be inadequately addressed—or so perceived. An incomplete assessment of the client's status and needs can result. Communication with the physician may also be strained if the case manager is merely a disembodied voice. The physician can view the telephonic case manager as the person who is going to deny or approve the treatment plan and therefore look upon the relationship as adversarial. When good rapport is possible, both the physician and the case manager can focus on the client and form a collaborative association.

3. The plan for home care may be inappropriate without actual assessment of the client's environment. For example, a client's discharge orders are for dressing changes to a draining ulcer on the right leg, to be carried out three times daily.

The nurse case manager has been informed by the hospital discharge planner that the client has been taught the appropriate technique for dressing changes. The nurse case manager coordinates delivery of the necessary supplies to the client's home. However, no one knows that the client's home is unkempt and dirty. If the nurse case manager had been aware of the environmental problems, she could have helped ensure that the dressing supplies would be kept in a clean area. Allowing the client to perform dressing changes in the existing environment may contaminate the supplies and result in reinfection to the area and nonhealing of the ulcer.

4. One person cannot have in-depth knowledge of all the sociocultural perspectives and lifestyles throughout the country. Speech patterns in one section of the country may be considered coarse and/or rude in other areas. The availability of community assistance varies among urban, suburban, and rural areas. Many isolated, rural, or farming communities rely on neighbor support for caretaking during illness as a way of life. Allowing strangers into the home as caretakers would be viewed negatively. In urban communities, neighbors acting as caretakers is not likely or expected. Since telephonic nurse case managers work with clients on a nationwide basis, this variation in cultural norms could result in miscommunication with the client and inappropriate coordination of care.

On-Site Case Management

On-site case management requires face-to-face interaction between the nurse case manager and the client. The initial client evaluation is performed either in the client's home or in the inpatient facility. The nurse case manager or rehab nurse may also attend physician follow-up appointments or outpatient therapy sessions with the client. If appropriate, the on-site case manager may conduct a job analysis at the place of employment or discuss development of a light- or modified-duty position. Of course, on-site visits and telephonic coordination of care are used as needed.

On-site can be the most costly case management for the insurance carrier. If appropriate case selection is achieved with an effective "red flag" system, the insurer can properly match case type and management strategy (telephonic or on-site). And the outcome is likely to be enhanced relationships among the health care team and the client, the most accurate and comprehensive evaluation, and greater savings through better planning as well as improved client satisfaction.

SKILLS SPECIFIC TO THE EXTERNAL NURSE CASE MANAGER

In general, the external nurse case manager or rehab nurse needs to perfect the same skills that the internal nurse case manager requires. (See Chapter 4 for details.) As a brief overview, the skills needed are as follows: communication, tact and diplomacy, assertiveness, collaboration, negotiation, marketing and networking, investigation, a sophisticated knowledge of nursing and pertinent law, critical thinking and problem solving, research, assessment, organization, prioritization, delegation, creativity, and self-discipline.

Most of these skills are interdependent. The nurse case manager with proficiency in one area will likely have superior ability in all areas. The following discussion focuses on negotiating, marketing, networking, and investigational skills. These skills are of special importance within the external case management context.

Negotiating Skills

The art of negotiating is arriving at a common goal between two or more people, pertaining to a common situation. Much of the work of the external nurse case manager involves negotiating for reduced costs with providers of services and extracontractual benefits with claims adjusters. For a client who was injured at work, negotiation skills will be paramount in discussing and recommending modified- or light-duty job positions. Negotiation skills and the negotiation process are neither inborn nor independent. The skills and process of negotiation can be learned and depend upon excellent communication skills, assertiveness, research skills, writing skills, and interpersonal relationships. Chapter 4 gave a brief description of the negotiation process. The four steps involved in negotiating will now be explored in greater depth.

The three knows

The first step is arriving at the answers to the "three knows," and this step begins before initial contact is made:

- *Know what it is.* If you are coordinating a service, know the exact nature of the service. For example, if you have received approval for 6 hours of nursing care, know the level of skill and amount of care that will be needed. Know the hours, days, and time limits that are involved. Know the home environment, presence or absence of family members, and other details that the provider might find helpful. If you are coordinating home durable medical equipment (DME), such as oxygen, know the equipment options and their differences. Have the physician's prescription regarding flow and know whether continuous or intermittent administration is necessary. Is the client ambulatory or bedridden? Will the client need portable oxygen? Are you renting or purchasing? Know the professional jargon of the provider. A nurse case manager unfamiliar with specific terminology may be perceived as inexperienced and unknowing and thus unable to defend client needs during the negotiation process. A case manager negotiating a modified job position with an employer must know the work environment, educational level and skills involved in various job duties, and the feasibility of developing a specific job. For example, it would not be appropriate to recommend that an employee be given a light-duty position of delivering mail for an employer equipped with an electronic mail delivery system.

- *Know who it is.* The nurse case manager should complete a comprehensive initial assessment of the client's status, needs, and home environment, prior to starting the negotiation process. Whether trying to persuade the carrier to approve extracontractual benefits or negotiating the cost of a service with a provider, the nurse case manager must be aware of all the details concerning the nursing, medical, psychosocial, environmental, financial, and spiritual needs of the client. As a simple example, coordinating the rental of an oversized wheelchair for an obese client who lives in a small, one-room apartment on the third floor of a building with no elevator would be an inappropriate and unsafe treatment option. Finding alternative, temporary living arrangements, with a family member if possible, would be more appropriate. Or—continuing with the client injured at work—if the case manager recommended a light-duty position of receptionist for a non-English speaking employee, the recommendation would be perceived as uninformed at best.

- *Know what it costs.* Contact a minimum of three providers to determine the average cost of services, equipment, or supplies in a specific area. When comparing rates, the comparison must be based on the identical item or service. Have model numbers and accessories or modifications requested. For example, the nurse case manager trying to find a wheelchair should be aware if the client will need elevating and removable leg rests and/or arm pieces. What kind of back and cushion is needed? Will a narrow or oversized chair be required? Will the item be a rental, rental to purchase, or out right purchase? Are there any service costs involved? In addition to knowing the cost of the item or service, the case manager must have a clear understanding of the policy benefits. Will the service or item be paid for at 100 percent? If not, how much will the client be responsible for out-of-pocket? What are the covered time limits for services or equipment?

For example, the nurse case manager coordinating outpatient physical therapy for a client should know how many physical therapy sessions are covered. If the covered benefit allows for a total of 30 outpatient physical therapy visits per year—or unlimited home care—it would behoove the nurse to coordinate home physical therapy, which will save transportation costs and be easier for the client. Knowledge of the contracts that the carrier already has in place and/or existing PPOs is extremely important in the negotiation process. Coordinating care for a client with a provider "out of network" is a waste of time and conveys a poor knowledge base.

Contacting the payer

After the case manager has the answers to the the three knows, she or he is ready to begin step 2 in the negotiating process, contacting the payer. The nurse case manager begins by discussing recommendations with the claims adjuster. If the recommendations fall within the benefit package, the case manager will request authorization to coordinate and implement the recommended care. If the recommendations are outside the usual contract, or "extracontractual," the nurse case manager must negotiate to persuade the claims adjuster that authorizing such care will be more cost-effective than staying within the scope of coverage. Since the case manager knows the details and the costs involved with both covered and alternative care options, he or she will be able to negotiate intelligently. For example, a nurse case manager worked with a client who had been admitted to a psychiatric hospital two to three times per year for the last 4 years. The average length of stay was 3 weeks, at a cost of approximately $17,000 per admission. The policy benefits covered inpatient care up to $50,000 annually. Outpatient benefits covered $50 per visit, with a maximum of 30 visits annually. After speaking with the client's physician, it was determined that if the client could receive outpatient treatment three times per week, the likelihood of hospital readmission would be greatly reduced. Through negotiation, the physician agreed to reduce his outpatient fee from $150/session to $110/session. The total cost per year would be $17,160.00, little more than one hospital admission. If the claims adjuster agrees to authorize the recommendation as extracontractual, and hospitalization is avoided, the carrier would save $32,840. When the case manager approached the claims adjuster with this recommendation, she was able to quote the history, cost of both the covered and extracontractual recommended treatment, and overall savings.

Contacting the provider

Once approval is received, the nurse case manager proceeds with step 3 in the negotiating process, contacting the provider. Both sides in the negotiation process are anxious to develop long-term relationships. Establishing good rapport, remaining flexible, and realizing that compromise is inherent in the negotiation process will produce the desired positive outcomes. The case manager should be knowledgeable and realistic about current costs and terms. For example, if the case manager has been quoted a cost of $35/hour for LPN care, requesting an hourly rate of $25 is inappropriate. Requesting $32/hour would be feasible if the case manager knows that several nursing agencies in the area charge similar rates. Knowledge of the average cost of a service or item is necessary so the case manager can begin negotiating at a realistic rate. High-mark-up items, such as infusion therapy, allow for more room for serious cost-cutting negotiation.

The outcome the case manager strives for is more than just arriving at the lowest cost. Low-cost home care and equipment with concomitant poor service or quality will likely be more costly in the long term. Cost-effectiveness must go hand in hand with good quality. For example, the nurse case manager who is coordinating 8 hours of RN care for a client contacts three nursing agencies. Agency "A" will provide the RN for $40/hour. Agency "B" and "C" will charge $43/hour. Agency "A" has a small RN staff and a poor reputation for filling all shifts. Agencies "B" and "C" have large RN staffs and excellent reputations for service. The nurse case manager who chooses agency "A" will undoubtedly receive frequent calls from the client complaining about unfilled shifts. The dissatisfied client will probably transfer his care to another agency, resulting in a waste of the case manager's time, no cost savings, and increased fragmentation of care. It should be emphasized that prior to the conclusion of any negotiations, the case manager must receive approval from the payer.

Documentation

The fourth step in the negotiation process, documentation, is as important as the actual negotiation. The nurse case manager must clearly document the results of the negotiation. Refer to Chapter 4 to review the letter-writing method of documenting, and the implications of incomplete documentation.

If the negotiation process involves coordinating services, equipment or supplies at a reduced rate, the nurse case manager must document the negotiated rate in correspondence to the provider. Succinct, accurate, descriptive terminology clearly defines negotiated terms. The original letter is forwarded to the provider, with a copy sent to the payer. (See Exhibit 6-1.)

Some case management companies offer bill review services as part of their contract with the insurance carriers. Since billing is often forwarded to a different department in the insurance company, the person receiving the bill may not be aware that case management services are involved and that the rates have been negotiated. Without this awareness the insurance carrier may inadvertently overpay. When a bill review system is in place, the provider submits the invoice directly to the case management company to ensure that the negotiated rate is the rate that is billed. If the invoice is correct, it is faxed to the insurance carrier for payment. If the rate is incorrect, the invoice is returned to the provider with an explanation. (See Exhibit 6-2.)

If the negotiation involves coordinating extracontractual benefits, this must be clearly stated in the case manager's report. As an illustration, use the example of the client who would benefit from extracontractual outpatient psychiatric treatment. The nurse case manager's

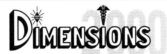

in Managed Care

Sandy Mandell, MA, CRRN, CIRS, CCM
DIRECTOR
201-882-3512

December 1, 19XX

Ms. Jan Smith
ABC Nursing Agency
111 East Main Street
Anywhere, USA 12345

Re: Client A

Dear Ms. Smith:

The XYZ Insurance Company has agreed to provide reimbursement for the following:

LPN level nursing care, from 8:00 AM to 4:00 PM, Monday through Friday

Start date: December 3, 19XX
End date: December 24, 19XX
Rate: $33.00/hour. There is no shift differential. There will be no additional charge for RN supervision or necessary RN supervisory visits. If there is an insufficient supply of LPNs for staffing and you find it necessary to substitute RN-level care, you will be reimbursed at the $33.00/hour LPN rate.

Sincerely,

[SIGNATURE]

Nurse Case Manager

cc: Claims Adjuster, XYZ Insurance Company

Exhibit 6-1. *Confirmation of provider services*

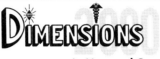

in Managed Care

Sandy Mandell, MA, CRRN, CIRS, CCM
DIRECTOR
201-882-3512

December 7, 19XX

Ms. Jan Smith
ABC Nursing Agency
111 East Main Street
Anywhere, USA 12345

Re: Client A

Dear Ms. Smith:
We are in receipt of bills submitted on the above named client for dates
of service as follows:

12/1/XX–12/7/XX   LPN-level care   8 hours/day

The bills are being returned for correction as outlined below:

The billed rate is for $35.00/hour. The negotiated rate, as per agreement
dated 12/1/XX, is $33.00/hour.

Please return the corrected bills to DIMENSIONS in Managed Care as
soon as possible so that prompt payment can be made by the insurance
carrier.

Sincerely,

[SIGNATURE]

Bill Review Dept.

cc: Claims Adjuster, XYZ Insurance Company

Exhibit 6-2.   *Provider bill review*

report would state, "With account approval, this consultant coordinated ongoing, outpatient psychiatric therapy for the client. Dr. X, the client's psychiatrist will treat the client three times weekly, at a negotiated rate of $110/session. Dr. X projects that increasing outpatient therapy will prevent hospital readmission. This consultant will contact Dr. X monthly to assess the client's status and progress."

In addition to documenting approval for extracontractual benefits in the report, many case management firms have designed alternative care proposals. These forms are completed by the nurse case manager and faxed to the claims adjuster for signature. The signed copy is then

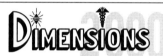

in Managed Care

Sandy Mandell, MA, CRRN, CIRS, CCM
DIRECTOR
201-882-3512

Insured: (name of client)   December 1, 19XX
Policy #: 1234567
SS #: 123-45-6789   Age: 38   Case Manager: Ms. Y

Diagnosis: Schizophrenia

Current Care: Limited outpatient psychotherapy. History of frequent hospitalization.

Cost: Approximately $17,000 per hospital stay

Alternative Care Recommendations: Outpatient psychotherapy three times weekly. Treating psychiatrist is Dr. X.

Cost: Negotiated rate of $110.00/session, or $330.00/week.

Savings: $32,840.00/year (if the client is not hospitalized).

Prognosis: Dr. X states that with additional outpatient therapy it is likely the client will not need inpatient treatment as frequently.

Proposed date of initiation of alternative care: 1/1/XX.

Frequency of a review during contract-exception period: monthly.

Authorized by: Date:

Exhibit 6-3.   *Alternative care proposal*

faxed back to the nurse case manager for her or his records (see Exhibit 6-3).

Marketing / Networking Skills

Nursing education does not generally include business courses covering strategies of marketing. However, as baccalaureate-prepared nurses increasingly fill positions of management or entrepreneurial ventures, knowledge of marketing and networking has become an integral part of their role. Nurses in general, and nurse case managers specifically, have been placed in a situation where self-education and "on-the-job-training" have had to take the place of a formal marketing background. Since many of the skills required for successful marketing are the same as those needed for case management, the nurse who chooses the role of marketer can be quite successful.

Unfortunately, people are not born with marketing expertise. Successful marketing involves knowing the art of negotiation, communication in all its forms, relating well with others, assertiveness, self-confidence, and initiative. In its broadest sense, marketing is the process of understanding and meeting someone else's needs. A relationship forms between a seller and a buyer, whereby the buyer will purchase an item or a service that is expected to improve the status quo. The seller persuades the buyer that his specific service or item is the highest quality and the most cost-effective. In case management the seller, or marketer, can be a nurse case manager selling case management services to insurance carriers, third-party administrators (TPAs), self-insured corporations, attorneys, unions and municipalities. Marketers are also found as providers of health care services, such as nursing agencies, rehabilitation institutes, and subacute facilities. Providers of equipment and supplies, such as surgical supply, pharmaceutical and respiratory companies, hire marketers to sell their products to nurse case managers as well as to various health care facilities.

A marketer without an audience is working in a vacuum. Inherent in the art of selling is developing and maintaining professional contacts and relationships. This is accomplished through networking. A network is a group of people who can support, inform, and guide. They are sources of prospective contacts for the marketer, and they provide resources and education for the buyer. Networks change over time and are composed of people from different backgrounds and with varying points of view. Professional networks are formed through joining various organizations, by attending seminars and conferences, and by forming alliances with other health care professionals. (See Appendix IV for a list of professional organizations.)

"Networking is the process of communicating with members of your network for the purpose of sharing resources and information."[6] Many independent nurse case managers, by virtue of their autonomy, do not have the professional camaraderie and support available to those working within a given facility. They can often feel isolated and detached especially when dealing with difficult situations or when problem solving. Social and professional networks within a facility help to resolve problems, establish feelings of unity, and offer emotional support. Independent nurse case managers can refine their networking skills and join various professional organizations to turn to when needed.

Networks are either horizontal or vertical. *Horizontal networks* are comprised of people of similar backgrounds who use the same professional jargon and maintain strong identification with the other members, for example, an organization for nurse case managers. *Vertical networks* are groups whose members are from diverse backgrounds, for example, the state nurses association, whose membership is drawn from varying levels of professionalism.[7] Another type of horizontal network is frequently found among case management and rehab nursing professional organizations. Membership often includes nurse case managers, insurance claims adjusters, various non-nursing health care professionals, and providers of services used by case managers. "Provider" members usually represent particular products or services. Nursing agencies, outpatient therapy facilities, transportation companies, surgical supply firms, and marketers for various rehabilitation and subacute facilities are only some of the professionals who might join such an organization.

The process of marketing case management has four essential steps: (1) learn every detail about the service or product; (2) create a marketing package, usually in the form of a brochure; (3) network and maintain positive professional relationships; and (4) persevere. Whether the marketer has a formal business background or is self-educated, the person who succeeds will be the one who believes in the service or product being sold, who has developed superior interpersonal relationship and creativity skills, and who remains sensitive to the needs of others.

Investigational Skills

The incidence of insurance fraud continues to escalate. People who commit fraud perceive the crime as nonviolent and victimless. This attitude absolves them from feelings of guilt and motivates additional fraud. In reality, everybody becomes a victim of fraud. Not only do the billions of dollars spent annually on fraudulent claims increase the cost of insurance premiums for everyone, but also treatment for the legitimately injured or ill person may be delayed owing to the growing cynicism among health care providers.

On-site rehab nurses, or nurse case managers, working with clients who have been injured at work or in motor vehicle accidents are frequently the first health care team members who suspect fraud or malingering. Although the rehab nurse is not employed as a detective per se, being alert to what may be fraudulent claims can lead to prompt investigation by appropriate professionals once initial investigation has been conducted.

The client who is a malingerer or who has filed a fraudulent claim may leave clues that should alert the attentive case manager to question further. For example, a new workers' compensation referral is received, with a client diagnosis of torn rotator cuff, right shoulder. The nurse case manager conducting her initial evaluation in the client's home notices that the living room is under construction and questions the client regarding the remodeling. Through effective assessment, interviewing and communication skills, and finesse, the case manager can determine if the client is continuing to do the remodeling himself, if he had begun it and is no longer able to continue since the injury, or if someone else is doing the work. If the client is working alone, it would be reasonable to suspect that the client is malingering. Other clues to malingering include grease under the client's fingernails, paint in the crevices of his skin, or other physical indicators that the client has recently been involved in strenuous activity.

Another frequently encountered situation involves the female employee with young school-age children who reports an injury during the summer months when school is out. Simple math may indicate that the amount of benefits received for a workers' compensation injury is greater than the client's regular salary minus the cost of child care. In this instance the incentive to remain out of work may be greater than that to return to work.

Client attitudes should also alert the case manager to look further. The client who speaks angrily about an employer, mistrusts the health care industry in general or the "deep pockets" of the insurance industry is more likely to feel that filing a fraudulent claim is an acceptable option. The client who has a strong religious belief system and feels like an essential employee is more likely to exhibit guilt about any dishonest behavior.

These scenarios alone do not constitute fraud. It is part of the nurse case manager's role to clarify information when fraud is suspected. Communicating with the client's physician, therapist, and employer will generate facts that will either reinforce or negate suspicion of fraudulent activity. If the employer states that the client is a valued employee, with an excellent attendance record and the therapist documents objective findings which are corroborated by the physician, the case manager probably misinterpreted certain details.

If, after clarifying the information, the nurse case manager still suspects that the client is a malingerer, various recommendations should be made to the insurance carrier or employer. A second opinion by an independent physician may be appropriate to establish whether the client is able to return to work. Encouraging the employer to design a light-duty position, such as sitting at a desk and answering the phone would in most instances force the client to return to work. Recommending surveillance (e.g., using the services of an investigation agency) is a last resort, since it is costly and time consuming and does not always elicit the desired results. Many times surveillance tapes clearly capture the client involved in strenuous activity, such as playing ball or shoveling snow. Unfortunately, when these tapes are brought to workers' compensation hearings (in those states that have them), the judge often rules that the client may have been feeling better on that day, which does not necessarily mean that he can return to physical labor 8 hours per day, 5 days per week.

The nurse case manager's documentation of objective findings is of great importance in detecting fraud. Documentation requires factual, nonjudgmental evidence, written clearly and succinctly. A detailed physical description of the client, including scars or tattoos and whether the client is usually clean-shaven, will assist with any additional investigative efforts by the insurance carrier. Many report formats include a section where the case manager can state subjective data, draw conclusions, and give opinions. Since the case management report may be discoverable (i.e., can be used in a lawsuit), subjective or speculative information should be discussed verbally, through telephone contact with the physicians, employer, and insurance carrier.

THE EXTERNAL NURSE CASE MANAGER IN THE MANAGED CARE SETTING

Several models of HMO managed care are in existence today. The medical group/independent physician association (MG/IPA) contracts with medical groups and independent physicians using a capitated rate. The medical group receives a predetermined and prepaid fee on a monthly basis. The group is then responsible for all diagnostic and treatment modalities. A second model used by HMOs is called the staff model, where the HMO owns and operates various health care facilities. Physicians and other staff members work directly for the HMO.[8]

All models of HMOs are increasing the use of case management. Kaiser Permanente, one of the largest HMOs, has been using case management since 1989. Case management within the HMO is viewed as a means of providing a more organized system to decrease costs. Although the job descriptions of case managers may vary from organization to organization, the goals of facilitating and coordinating cost-effective care remain constant.

Most case managers working for managed care organizations perform the role telephonically and provide utilization review and utilization management services. Other job functions may include assisting the client to access care that is not covered in the benefit package. For example, the case manager may refer the patient to government-funded programs and provide assistance in filling out various applications. Another role of the case manager working for an HMO is acting as "gatekeeper," which entails being responsible for coordinating care within the HMO system.

Some case managers working for managed care organizations do on-site visits. Examples include Health Service Operations in Pittsburgh, PA and Group Health Cooperative in the state of Washington. Both of these HMOs employ case managers to visit patients and families to coordinate appropriate care within the system and to design alternative care plans for necessities that the HMO does not provide.[9]

Another role of the nurse case manager working for an HMO involves participation in the development of provider networks, such as physical therapists, nursing agencies, equipment vendors, and the like. Managed care organizations enter into exclusive contracts with these providers, meaning insured members may only go to those who are "within network." Although some larger HMOs may use regional contractors who develop the provider network, the in-house case manager has input in the development process. The case manager has had extensive experience with numerous providers in the area. Her or his knowledge base and recommendations are highly regarded by the local or regional contractors.[10]

Much of the managed care philosophy is based on proactive care and prevention. The role of the case manager in managed care involves assessing the high-risk patient population and coordinating and monitoring care within the restrictions of the benefits, prior to large dollar expenditures. This role involves a high degree of creativity and problem solving. The nurse case manager's goal as patient advocate, gatekeeper, and facilitator is to balance appropriate and timely care in a cost-effective manner while remaining within the benefits and restrictions of the HMO coverage.

THE EXTERNAL NURSE CASE MANAGER IN THE INDEMNITY INSURANCE SETTING

Many traditional indemnity insurance companies use case management as a means of ensuring that high-quality and appropriate care is rendered in a cost-effective manner. Although the role of the case manager in managed care is similar, the indemnity insurance-based case manager works with a broader spectrum of choices and more flexibility within the benefit package. Traditional indemnity carriers now contract with provider networks as a means of holding down costs. However, the traditional indemnity carrier cannot require that the patient use a specific provider.

The role of the case manager within the traditional insurance industry may vary from one carrier to another; however, the basic job description remains generic (see Table 6-1). The general purpose of case management remains coordination of quality care for the high-dollar or serious claims in a cost-effective manner. The goal is to minimize fragmentation of care and to maximize utilization of services.

Each carrier establishes criteria to select clients who should be case managed. The criteria generally relate to either reaching a certain dollar threshold for a claim or having a specific diagnosis (for example, all clients with spinal cord injuries). A case manager who determines that a client would benefit from case management services contacts the client to assess his status and needs. Although health insurance case managers primarily use telephonic case management, some will conduct on-site visits when deemed necessary. Alternatively, workers' compensation case managers most frequently

Table 6-1. Typical job description of the case manager employed by an insurance company

PURPOSE OF THIS POSITION

Provide medical case management services to clients who have serious or high-dollar illness or injury. The health care coordinator assists in managing health care dollars while contributing to the quality health care services to minimize fragmentation in the delivery of health care to clients.

NATURE AND SCOPE

This position is essential to achieving the clinical services mission of providing comprehensive medical case management to clients utilizing medical expertise. The incumbent who reports to the clinical services/case management supervisor has the autonomy to coordinate quality health care services to minimize fragmentation in the delivery of health care to clients.

PRINCIPAL RESPONSIBILITIES

Determine need for case management intervention through gathering of relevant data and assessment of treatment, prognosis, resource utilization, and cost management.

Select cases for management where client outcome and/or liability can be positively influenced by telephonic or on-site case management for major disease categories and high dollar cases.

Interview, research, and gather information in order to formulate a case management plan in collaboration with the client and family and treatment team, identifying short- and long-term goals and process for meeting goals.

Demonstrate knowledge and understanding of client's diagnosis, prognosis, care needs and outcome goals of the treatment/care plan.

Demonstrate understanding of cost containment strategies regardless of limitations of policy/benefits available to the client.

Empower client to make appropriate decisions by providing education and resources.

Monitor quality of care, service, and products delivered to client to determine if goals are being achieved.

Maintain rapport and communication with client, family, and treatment team.

Evaluate methodology designed to measure client's response to health care services and products, appropriateness of providers' plan of care, and quality of products and services.

Document case management activity, which includes the rationale for decisions, alternatives, and treatment options using established computer system guidelines.

Assist in the identification of alternative treatment plans to facilitate appropriate care and cost-effective outcomes.

Comply with the established case management standards of practice.

Serve as a client advocate.

OTHER RESPONSIBILITIES

Practice within the scope of licensure and/or certification

Act in accordance with laws and procedures regarding client confidentiality and release of information.

Participate in health care coordinator orientation and education.

Provide case management orientation and education to internal and external customers.

Research and identify quality external medical care management services when necessary. Review, supervise, and monitor treatment options proposed by external case manager.

Correlate insurance concepts with case management principles.

Review case management claims as necessary.

Serve as a medical resource to internal and external customers.

Represent health care by participation in professional, industry, and community organizations.

Maintain continuing education appropriate to the practice of case management.

Other duties as assigned.

(With permission from Time Insurance Co.)

use on-site case management because on-site is more sensitive to detecting malingering or fraud. This also facilitates the goal of returning the worker to the job as quickly as possible. If the insurance carrier does not have personnel to carry out on-site case management, it contracts with independent case management firms to perform the on-site case management services.

Review of the literature indicates that there is no universal model of case management for the insurance industry. Although all insurance carriers strive to minimize their costs, many carriers do not implement case management effectively. Many insurance-based case managers coordinate, implement, and document, but have no defined plan of care. The case management focuses on applying disease-specific treatment protocols that may not be individualized to a specific patient. Without using a comprehensive approach to case management, the likelihood of fragmentation of care and inappropriate or delayed treatment increases. When using a carefully designed plan, the dual advocacy roles of the nurse case manager are enhanced. The case manager is not only responsible for identifying required services but also for understanding "the bottom line." Since most insurance companies are public, for-profit corporations, increasing profits by decreasing cost is an essential aspect of coordinating care. Because of this, the case manager may have difficulty when recommending extracontractual benefits to the decision makers in the benefits department. If the case manager can outline a clear plan of care, documenting rationale and projected outcomes, the people in the benefits department will be more likely to approve expenses not ordinarily required. A comprehensive approach to case management will allow for simplification of identifying needs, smoother coordination of care, and increased patient satisfaction.

Since the insurance-based case manager works within the confines of a specific carrier, documentation of activities is ordinarily computerized. Usually, just a short entry by date is necessary. If a new case manager assumes the responsibility for a given client, the complete history and past recommendations with outcomes are easily accessible in the computer data base.

THE CASE MANAGER AS INDEPENDENT CONTRACTOR

Many nurse case managers in the insurance industry are not employed directly by an insurance company. Instead, they are employed by or have their own rehabilitation and/or case management firms. Independent case management companies receive referrals from the insurance company and manage cases as representatives of the carrier.

Many aspects of an independent case manager's job are similar to that of the insurance-based case manager. The goals of coordinating timely and appropriate care in a cost-effective manner remain constant. The emphasis on quality and defragmentation is the same. However, there are several differences in the work performed by the case manager employed by an insurance carrier and by the independent nurse case manager, as follows:

1. The insurance-based case manager may have some discretionary power within the covered population of the company to direct case management services to those who would most benefit. The case manager also makes the decision for discontinuing case management services. The independent case manager receives most referrals from insurance carriers. Although early referral is encouraged, an insurance company case manager may not place clients with an independent case manager in a timely fashion. Independent case managers often deal with client referrals whose *date of loss* (the date of injury or diagnosis) is several years old. The independent case manager may recommend discontinuing the client from case management services because the patient is stable, has reached maximum medical improvement (MMI), and/or has returned to work and no longer needs coordinated services. However if the insurance carrier case manager disagrees, the decision of the insurance carrier will prevail.

2. The insurance-based case manager has the autonomy to approve recommendations that are within the scope of the benefit package. The independent case manager must receive authorization from the insurance carrier prior to implementing care.

3. The insurance-based case manager uses a nursing care plan format and does not make formal reports. The independent

case manager must generate comprehensive reports every 30 days, with recommendations for continued care. The reports are mailed to the insurance carrier. (See samples of reports in Appendix I.)

4.   Independent nurse case managers function in dual advocacy roles. Although they are patient advocates, they also represent the insurance carrier and must always remain cognizant of covered benefits and cost. Usually the independent case manager documents savings either in monthly or quarterly reports. Since the insurance carrier is paying for the independent case management services, it is imperative that savings be clearly documented.

5.   A major problem for independent case managers is an inability to follow up. The insurance-based case manager usually discontinues case management services when the client reaches the point of recovery in the sometimes mistaken belief that it is too costly to maintain case management services if the client has reached medical stability. However, if the client has a relapse or has difficulty adjusting to life changes, continued case management would allow for expedient, efficient and cost-effective care. Therefore, the independent case manager must be able to promote the benefits of maintaining short-term follow-up case management services.

When assisting a client injured in a work-related accident, the case manager is usually directed to discontinue services when the physician releases the client to return to work. Such early closure may lead to fragmented care, a relapse, or exacerbation of the injury, resulting in continued payment of benefits to the injured worker. For example, an injured worker may return to work for a day or a week and determine that he or she is unable to perform his or her job duties. The worker returns to the physician, resumes medical treatment, and remains out of work. If the case manager had been allowed to follow up, this situation would be known immediately. Contacting the physician to determine the client's abilities and disabilities, the nurse case manager can then help the employer design a temporary, light or modified position. Or through an independent medical exam or vocational counseling, the case manager could assist the client to a successful return to work. The independent medical exam provides an objective, second assessment of the client's abilities. Vocational counseling will help define appropriate work responsibilities for the client and is useful to the employer in designing modified positions. Long-term and effective cost savings generated through case management depend on continuation of services through completion of care.

Regardless of the setting, the role of the external case manager is to coordinate efficient, effective care in a manner satisfactory to both client and carrier. When collaboration, creativity, and autonomy are successfully combined, the injured or ill client will return to a productive lifestyle or achieve the maximum level of functioning.

PRIVATE PRACTICE CASE MANAGEMENT

A small but growing area in case management is private practice case managers who are hired by and work directly for the client. Most clients are elderly, unable to coordinate necessary equipment, supplies, or home care. Their difficulties may result from Medicare or supplemental insurance restrictions, lack of information or decreased ability to function. Often, referrals come from family members desperate for assistance in coordinating appropriate, cost-effective care for their elderly relatives.

With advances in health care technology, the average lifespan has increased. It is no longer rare for the middle-aged population to be "sandwiched" between caring for their children, and for their aging parents. Placement of a parent in a nursing home is often inappropriate, undesirable, or too costly. Alternative care options may not be known or available. The Medicare system is bureaucratic, often confusing, and ambiguous. Rigid restrictions limit the amount of care available.

A growing group of entrepreneurial, creative case managers are marketing their services to this population. The case manager assists the client or family member in designing alternative care options, coordinating appropriate care, assisting with filing of claims and reducing out-of -pocket costs.

THE FUTURE OF EXTERNAL CASE MANAGEMENT

Projecting the future of a profession during times of profound change is difficult at best. However, certain indicators appear universal in the rapidly changing health care arena. Managed care, an integrated delivery system, an emphasis on prevention, and the need for quality combined with cost-effectiveness will continue to shape the evolution of the health care system and of case management.

The job of the traditional nurse case manager, responsible for piecemeal negotiation of the cost of care, is disappearing. Documented cost savings based on provider discounts cannot be accomplished in a world of provider networks, contracts, and capitated and bundled rates. Since capitation is a monthly fee paid to a physician per insured life, regardless of the amount of care delivered, the less care that is delivered, the higher the physician's profits. Historically, the physician who prescribed the most diagnostic exams and performed the most procedures produced the highest profits. In addition, bundled rates, predetermined costs based on a diagnosis, mean that a client with a given diagnosis will be worth X amount of dollars to a physician to cover all expenses related to that person's care. Such fee structuring has negated the case manager's traditional role of negotiating provider cost.

The traditional case manager used to collaborate with the physician and coordinate the least expensive care that would meet client needs. With the explosion of managed care and rigid restrictions for length of hospital stay, the physician has lost much autonomy concerning patient disposition and discharge. Insurance companies can now restrict the scope and intensity of care available by offering only narrow coverage options. Much of the economic "fat" has already been trimmed from the system. The focus of external case managers will change, focusing on maintaining the health of designated groups through disease management programs.

The nurse case manager of the future will be a highly educated, well-spoken and well-informed specialist within a specific area of health care. The minimum level of preparation will be at the baccalaureate or master's level. Certification will be a requisite, as will be continuing education. Business savvy and extensive knowledge of the insurance industry and managed care will be essential. Creativity, assertiveness, and interpersonal relationship and leadership skills will be necessary components for the case manager to succeed.

The future case manager will be computer literate by necessity and able to use highly technical databases for appropriate and cost-effective coordination of care. Some high-tech products and services are already being used by case managers in rural areas as alternative and cost-effective options to emergency room visits and cardiac rehabilitation, as the following examples show:

> CallDoctor Inc. in San Diego is a franchised, mobile physician treatment center. "An emergency room on wheels,"[11] Call-Doctor can treat nonthreatening emergencies at home. According to Dr. Grehsham Bayne, the chairman of CallDoctor, "90 percent of people seen in America's emergency rooms do not have life-threatening illnesses."[12]

> Transtelephonic Exercise Monitoring (TEM) gives patients in rural areas who need cardiac rehabilitation an alternative option. Rather than travel a long distance to a hospital exercise program, the client carries out the exercise program at home. Through electrodes applied to the chest, a head set and a small device worn on a belt, the patient's electrocardiogram (EKG) and voice are transmitted through a modem to a nurse who monitors the exercise program.

As technology continues to connect people through computer software, the role of the case manager will become broader. Alternative care options will be more diverse and will require intensive patient teaching. The nurse case manager coordinating high-tech home care will need to understand thoroughly the product or service and be able to assess the difference between the high-quality service provider and the charlatan.

Case management of the future will be proactive rather than re-active. The goals of case management will be prevention and increased quality. The population served by the independent case manager will be the well, but at risk, rather than the acutely ill or injured. High-risk individuals will be managed prior to the onset of an illness. The term *case management* may even evolve into *prevention management*.

Disease management programs, a new twist on patient-centered health care, are beginning to flourish. Although there are many kinds of disease management programs, the generally accepted definition is a "comprehensive and coordinated system of care that manages a disease state, rather than an acute episode."[13] Most disease management programs are designed for the person with self-managing, chronic illness, such as asthma or diabetes. Both diseases have costly and multiple complications. With appropriate patient education, coordination of care and resource referrals, many of the complications can be avoided or delayed.

The case manager's future role will include identification of those patients who are at risk for acute exacerbation of an illness. Sophisticated information systems will enable the case manager to identify such high-risk populations, as well as the clinical triggers for chronic illnesses. Once identified, the case manager will contact the client to conduct a comprehensive assessment of needs. Through extensive data gathering and collaborative efforts, disease management programs will be developed, implemented, and monitored. The nurse case manager will play a central role in the disease management process.

The case manager of the future will be part of provider networks and will be reimbursed on a shared risk or capitated basis. Just as the solo physician practice is becoming endangered, independent case managers will no longer be able to survive as single entities. The independent case management firm will be a central part of a larger group of providers. Partnership marketing will replace the usual sales methods. Case managers will have to form partnerships with their customers so that both are working towards resolving a common problem, rather than one person selling a service to another.[14]

As managed care, physician alliances, and integrated health care become entrenched in the delivery system, and as the focus of health care continues the shift towards prevention, the opportunities for case management will increase. The role may broaden and/or take on a different shape, but the need for coordination of time-effective, cost-effective, high-quality care will remain at the hub of health care.

Chapter Highlights

* External case management developed as a strategy to control the cost of care associated with catastrophic illness and injury.
* The major approach to cost control is to reduce hospital length of stay and use the least expensive level of appropriate care. Utilization review and utilization management processes facilitate achieving these goals.
* External case management is practiced telephonically and/or on-site.
* Case managers in all settings must possess a range of social and communication skills. In addition, the external case manager needs to perfect skill in negotiation, marketing and networking, and investigation.
* External case managers work for managed care organizations, for indemnity insurance companies, as independent contractors representing insurance carriers, and as entrepreneurs in private practice.
* The external case manager collaborates with the internal case manager and other health care providers to coordinate cost-effective care across the continuum, with smooth transitions from one level to another, and to design alternative care proposals when appropriate.
* When working with clients injured at work, the external case manager works collaboratively with physicians and employers to assist with a timely return to work.
* The role of the external case manager is evolving to a more proactive approach with a focus on prevention, education, and alternative treatment.

1. Erkel, E.(1993, Jan.). The impact of case management in preventive services. *Journal of Nursing Administration.* 23(1), 27.

2. Pueraro, M.(speaker) (1995, Jan. 20). Case management: What it is, what it isn't. National Association of Rehabilitation Professionals in the Private Sector. West Conshohocken, PA.

3. Schaffer, C. (1995, Jan.–Feb.). Case management's role in networks. *Continuing Care.* 14(1), 21.

4. Pueraro, Case management.

5. Ibid.

6. Hamilton, M. (1996). *Realities of contemporary nursing.* (2d ed.). Menlo Park, CA: Addison-Wesley. p. 355.

7. Hein, E., & Nicholson, M.(1986). *Contemporary leadership behavior: selected readings.* (2d ed.). Boston MA: Little Brown. p. 190.

8. Blodgett, C. (1992, July–Aug.–Sept.). HMO case management: Medical group model. *The Case Manager.* 3(3), 35.

9. Gerson, V. (1995, Jan.–Feb.–Mar.). HMO case management. *The Case Manager.* 6(1), 79–88.

10. Ibid., 86–88.

11. Bayne, G. (1995, April). When off road is better. *Case Management Advisor.* (6)4, 47.

12. Ibid.

13. Todd, W. (1995, June). New mindsets in asthma: interventions and disease management. *The Journal of Care Management.* 1(1), 37.

14. Repecky, P. (1995, April). Find, persuade key buyers of CM services; Here's how. *Case Management Advisor.* 6(4), 55.

The External Case *Management Process*

Nurse case managers working outside health facilities in the places where care is rendered are referred to as *external case managers*. The process of external case management closely parallels the nursing process but is more global. The external case management process does not include hands-on nursing. It does incorporate the additional components of case selection, multidisciplinary assessment, collective planning, coordinating, negotiating, and evaluating the outcomes in terms of cost and quality, as well as client status. In addition to assisting the client with health care needs, the external case management process includes vocational, motivational, and financial strategies.

This chapter examines the case management process from the perspective of the external case manager or any case manager working outside a health care facility. Upon completion of this chapter you will be able to answer the following questions:

1. How is the case management process different from the nursing process?
2. How do the two major models of external case management compare?
3. How does the case manager receive referrals of new clients?
4. How does the focus of the case manager differ according to the referral source?

5.   What are the stages of the case management process?
6.   What is the responsibility of the case manager during each stage of the case management process?

MODELS OF THE EXTERNAL CASE MANAGEMENT PROCESS

In the evolution of professional nursing practice, case management is still in its infancy. The concept of case management continues to become entrenched in health care and is increasingly accepted as the necessary focal point in managing complex care within a fragmented, multidimensional, and opaque system. With growth and experience, a clearly defined and structured process continues to develop.

In 1991, the National Task Force on Case Management, founded by representatives from 36 professional associations, presented a definition of case management along with a comprehensive case management model (see Figure 7-1). The National Task Force's definition is: "Case Management is a collaborative process which assesses, plans, implements, coordinates, monitors and evaluates options for services to meet an individual's health needs through communication and available resources to promote quality, cost-effective outcomes."[1]

The model uses advocacy, collaboration, problem solving, and communication as specific strategies to establish a balance among the consumer and family, the provider, and the payer. The strategies are accomplished through the processes of assessment, planning, facilitating, coordinating, and evaluating.[2]

This model, although accurately depicting the cyclical nature of case management, omits some basic and essential areas of the process: documentation, implementation, and reevaluation. Those three segments are what differentiate the case management process from the nursing process. In addition, the National Task Force model considered advocacy as a *strategy* (a method by which something is achieved). We consider advocacy as part of the *role* (a persona internalized by the case manager as part of the job). One other part

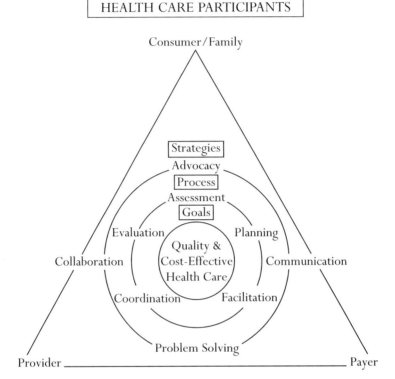

Figure 7-1. *Model of case management (National Task Force on Case Management)*

of the model that may indicate fragmentation is the apparent lack of communication between the payer and the provider.

Because of the shifting role of the case manager, as well as the need for a comprehensive and future-oriented model, Kathy Hruz, RN, BSN, CCM, designed a case management model in 1995 based on a systems approach to the nursing process (see Figure 7-2). Essentially, Hruz's model represents a process of assessment, data collection, data analysis, and identification of needs. Once the needs are identified, goals, outcomes, and projected time frames are assessed. At this point in the process a case management plan is developed.

To achieve a realistic and operative plan, a comprehensive, accurate assessment involves the use of various strategies within the process. These strategies include (1) prioritization of needs; (2) identification

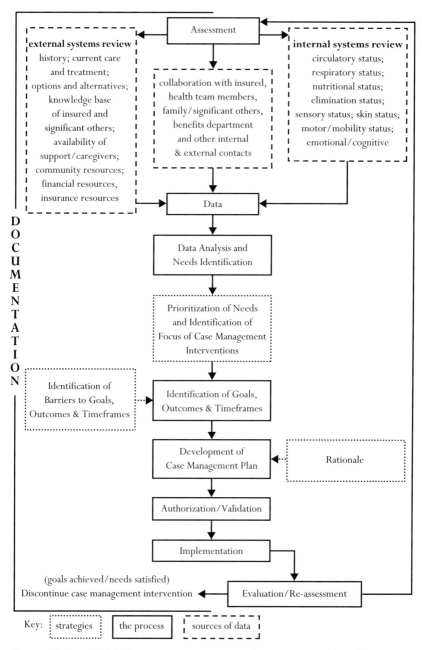

Figure 7-2. *Model of case management process (systems approach) with permission from Kathy Hruz, RN, BSN, CCM*

of barriers present to determine appropriate goals, outcomes and time frames; and (3) a clear and concise rationale that supports the appropriateness of the suggested plan of care.

Once the case management plan is complete, the case manager must verify the insurance benefits and request authorization to proceed with implementation. The plan is reviewed with the client, since participation in the planning process empowers the client and brings up any unforeseen impediments. Evaluation, reevaluation, and reassessment are ongoing and continuous as the client's status changes. Documentation is carried out during each step of the process.

As with the insurance-based case manager, a universal model for the independent case manager does not exist. However, most rehab and case management companies follow a general model similar to Hruz's model of assessment, collaboration, identification of needs, development of a plan of care, authorization, coordination, implementation, and evaluation.

Because of this lack of a universally accepted case management model, many case managers today bring to their practice their own unique styles. Personality plays as much a part in determining the process as does the current research, both empirical and scientific. There is a great need for additional research in this area. Through analysis of outcomes and the design of an appropriate model, the process of case management will be enhanced in its goals of decreasing fragmentation, decreasing the cost of health care, and increasing quality across the continuum.

THE REFERRAL

The case management process begins with the referral. The case manager working for an insurance company determines which clients would benefit from case management services based on either a diagnosis or a predetermined dollar amount. The insurance case manager may directly manage the client's care telephonically and/or on-site, or may contact an independent case management firm to provide the necessary services.

If an independent contractor is contacted, the insurance company case manager may indicate issues that he or she wants addressed, limits on services provided, and/or goals to be met. The referral usually includes basic information about those providers that the case manager will be contacting for the client's care (see Exhibit 7-1).

Workers' Compensation Referrals

Case managers working with clients injured in work-related accidents must have extensive knowledge about orthopedics and neurology. The vast majority of injuries occurring at work involve the low back, rotator cuff tears, knee injuries, and/or injuries resulting from repetitive activities, such as carpal tunnel syndrome. The experienced case manager working with such clients must know where to find the necessary specialists, rehabilitation settings, and therapy facilities.

The case manager must be thoroughly grounded in the workers' compensation laws for the state in which the person was injured. Unlike group health insurance—where the specific benefit package dictates the extent of coverage, regardless of where the patient lives—the limits and extent of workers' compensation coverage are set by the workers' compensation commission of each state, and the guidelines vary from state to state. These differences affect the case manager's recommendations, activities, and goals. In some states, such as New York, the injured person has the right to choose the treating physician. However, New York guidelines also include a physician fee schedule: The physician cannot charge the patient more than the allowed amount. Thus the patient's doctor of choice may refuse to treat the patient filing under workers' compensation because of the low reimbursement rate. Across the river, in New Jersey, the employer is free to choose the treating physician. When case management is involved, the employer will usually defer the choice of physicians to the case manager. Since a fee schedule does not exist in New Jersey, the case manager can assign treatment to the best physician within a specific specialty area.

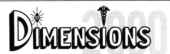

in Managed Care

Sandy Mandell, MA, CRRN, CIRS, CCM
DIRECTOR
201-882-3512

DIARY DATE: _____
DIMENSIONS # _____

REFERRAL

DATE: _____   CONSULTANT: _____
PHONE: _____   FAX: _____

INSURED: _____   ACCOUNT: _____
ADDRESS: _____   ADDRESS: _____
PHONE: _____   FAX: _____ PHONE_____
                               CONTACT PERSON:
                               _____

POLICY #: _____
DOB: _____ DOL: _____ SS#: _____
DIAGNOSIS: _____
PHYSICIAN: _____   ATTORNEY: _____
ADDRESS: _____   ADDRESS: _____
_____   _____
PHONE: _____ FAX: _____   PHONE: _____ FAX: _____
EMPLOYER: _____   OCCUPATION: _____
ADDRESS: _____
PHONE: _____   FAX: _____
THERAPIST: _____
ADDITIONAL CONTACTS: _____
_____
_____

REQUEST FOR: WC _____ GH _____ MVA _____ EVAL-ONE _____
INSTRUCTIONS:

Exhibit 7-1.   *Case management referral*

Another important difference between workers' compensation and medical insurance is the responsibility of the workers' compensation carrier to reimburse lost wages as well as to cover all medical costs. Although wage replacement limits vary across the country, all insurers and self-funded employers are mandated to reimburse both medical costs and some predetermined percentage of salary. In addition, statistics indicate that "if an injured worker is not back to work within six months of injury, there is only a 50 percent chance that he will return."[3] Furthermore, if the claimant has not returned within a year, the return to work rate drops to 25 percent, and to almost zero after 2 years out of work.[4] Often, the injured workers have adjusted to a lower standard of living or have found other employment where they are paid "under the table." The incentive to return to work drops in proportion to the period of time out of work. Since wage replacement is often more costly to the insurance carrier than medical costs, many carriers' primary goal is to achieve a timely return to work.

A third difference between traditional indemnity health insurance and workers' compensation insurance is the independent medical exam (IME). Although this varies from state to state, many workers' compensation carriers require an IME (similar to a second opinion) before authorizing expensive procedures or diagnostic tests. Physicians who perform IMEs presumably do not gain much from this review. This is especially true in states where a physician performing an IME can never be used to treat the patient. As an example, if a person was injured at work, and sustained a low back injury, the treating physician may recommend a laminectomy. Either the carrier or the case manager would schedule an IME with a board-certified orthopedist and forward all medical records for the physician to review. The case manager may, or may not attend this appointment. The IME physician examines the patient and renders an opinion regarding the appropriateness of a laminectomy. If the IME physician recommends 6 weeks of conservative treatment, such as physical therapy, prior to considering a surgical procedure, the carrier will in all likelihood deny the treating physician approval to operate. After 6 weeks of therapy, if the claimant continues to complain of pain, and the treating physician continues to recommend a laminectomy, a second IME would be scheduled.

Another important aspect of workers' compensation versus medical insurance is the litigious nature of compensation claims. Although not all claimants hire an attorney and not all states require attorney authorization, there are occasions when this is the case. When the case manager receives a referral, the claimant's attorney must be contacted before contacting the claimant. The case manager corresponds with the attorney and encloses a blank consent form, which the claimant will be asked to sign (see Exhibits 7-2 and 7-3).

Although there are many legitimate reasons for legal representation, there are an equal number of attorneys with hidden agendas. Unfortunately, the attorney who wants to increase the cost of the claim (so that the attorney fee will be higher) may deny case management services or demand so many restrictions that the case manager is incapable of assisting the claimant to achieve the best possible medical care and a timely return to work. When this occurs, it is a lose-lose situation for everyone except the attorney. Once all the preliminary approvals are received, the case manager forwards a letter to the claimant explaining that a case manager will contact him or her to schedule an appointment (See Exhibit 7-4).

During this first appointment, data are collected for a complete, comprehensive initial assessment (see Chapter 4 for review of the assessment process). If the initial evaluation is scheduled to take place at the physician's office, the case manager will discuss the treatment plan, time frames, and estimated return-to-work date. The case manager must also speak with the physician about any preexisting conditions, exacerbation of preexisting conditions, the relationship of the patient's complaints to the work injury, and the possibility of malingering or fraud. If a preexisting condition has been exacerbated, the carrier is reimbursed a percentage of costs through a state fund set up specifically for this type of claim.

Following the client's initial evaluation and discussion with the physician, the case manager will contact all other providers who have been or will be treating the claimant, such as therapists or

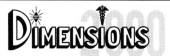

in Managed Care

Sandy Mandell, MA, CRRN, CIRS, CCM
DIRECTOR
201-882-3512

Attorney   Date
Re: Claim #:   DIMENSIONS #:

Dear

DIMENSIONS in Managed Care has been asked by _____ Insurance Co., to have a nurse case manager/rehabilitation specialist assist in
the coordination of medical care for your client. We have found that by
having a rehabilitation nurse work with the injured person, medical care
leads to a speedier recovery, due to more timely treatment intervention.
Please note that the rehabilitation specialist does not get involved with
any liability issues and will not in any way be discussing that aspect.

A rehabilitation specialist will be contacting you for authorization to meet
with your client. Enclosed with this letter is a copy of a consent that your
client will be asked to sign. This is needed in order for the rehabilitation
specialist to gather important medical information necessary for assisting
in your client's care.

If you need more information or have any questions, please feel free to
contact me.

Sincerely

[SIGNATURE]

Exhibit 7-2.   *Sample letter to attorney*

nursing agencies. The case manager will then contact the claimant's
employer to assess the claimant's job description, the possibility of
a temporary or permanent light-duty position, or other available
positions where comparable or transferable skills could be used.

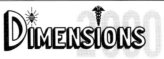

in Managed Care

Sandy Mandell, MA, CRRN, CIRS, CCM
DIRECTOR
201-882-3512

NAME _____ DATE _____

I hereby authorize the representative of DIMENSIONS in Managed Care to be permitted to review and obtain copies of all hospital, medical, and other related records and to discuss pertinent information with professionals involved in my care. I understand that all information released will be handled confidentially, in compliance with the Federal Privacy Act and the Federal Alcohol and Drug Abuse Act.

I also understand that I may revoke this authorization at any time by written, dated communication to the releasing agency or hospital. Copies of this consent are considered valid.

_____
Signature of client

_____   _____
Signature of witness   Signature of family member,
                                     (if client unable to sign—or if
                                     client a minor)

Exhibit 7-3. *Release of information*

After the case manager has gathered all pertinent information, a plan of care is developed with the dual goals of a timely return to work and maximum medical improvement (MMI). Recommended activities will depend upon the specific state workers' compensation guidelines. The case manager then contacts the carrier case manager, or insurance adjuster, to review the recommended activities. If the carrier agrees, the case manager will receive approval to continue with the process.

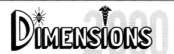

in Managed Care

Sandy Mandell, MA, CRRN, CIRS, CCM
DIRECTOR
201-882-3512

Client   Date:
CLAIM #:
DIMENSIONS #:

Dear Ms. Kahn:

DIMENSIONS in Managed Care has been retained by Total Health Insurance Co., your insurance carrier regarding your workers' compensation injury.

Your file has been assigned to Ms. King, a rehabilitation nurse who will be assisting in the coordination of your medical care and treatment.

Ms. King will be contacting you by phone to arrange for an appointment in order to discuss your needs.

Sincerely,

[SIGNATURE]

Teresa Kowalski, RN, CCM

cc: Erik Scott, adjuster—Total Health Insurance Co.

Exhibit 7-4. *Introduction letter to the client injured at work*

Motor Vehicle Insurance Referrals

The process for case managers working with clients injured in motor vehicle accidents is similar to that of workers' compensation. Varying state laws dictate what is or is not covered. The insurance carrier has the right to schedule independent medical exams (IMEs) prior to approving recommended procedures. The litigious nature of motor vehicle accidents requires attorney contact.

In contrast to workers' compensation, the injured person must pay an annual deductible out-of-pocket. In addition, many states have placed a cap on motor vehicle insurance coverage. If a person is injured in a motor vehicle accident in a state with such a cap, that amount of medical expenses will be paid by the motor vehicle insurance (after the deductible is met). After that amount has been reached, depending on the type of policy the person chose, additional medical care will be paid by the person's health insurance carrier.

Health Insurance Referrals

Case management for clients with traditional indemnity health insurance is voluntary on the part of the client. When the case manager receives a referral from the insurance company, a letter is forwarded to the client explaining the purpose of case management and its voluntary nature. (See Exhibit 7-5.)

In contrast to workers' compensation insurance, the case manager working with health insurance does not need attorney approval and is not restricted to state-mandated guidelines. She or he can be much more creative with planning care (within the limits of the benefit package).

Since the insurance company is not paying lost wages, a timely return to work or available light duty are not issues. During the course of information gathering, the employer is not contacted. Although the case managers view their role as the patient's advocates and want to assist the patient holistically, they must remain aware that they are representing—and being paid by—the insurance carrier. The case manager working within the insurance company will not want to reimburse the external case manager for time spent on issues for which the carrier is not responsible.

Another difference in the case management process between health insurance and workers' compensation is the need to attend most physician appointments with the client. When working with a client insured with health insurance, the case manager rarely

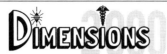

in Managed Care

Sandy Mandell, MA, CRRN, CIRS, CCM
DIRECTOR
201-882-3512

Client   Date:
POLICY #:
DIMENSIONS #:

Dear Mr. Lopez:

As representatives of Triangle Insurance Company, we have become aware of your health problem from our claims office and are certain this must be a difficult time for you and your family.

We have many services available to you through DIMENSIONS in Managed Care and have arranged for a nurse case manager to contact you to discuss how she might be able to assist you during this time.

Please be assured that this voluntary program is designed to help you obtain the best and most appropriate health care services, as well as preserve your benefit dollars. There is no cost to you for this service.

Sincerely,

[SIGNATURE]

Dayna Romero, RN, CCM

cc: Tanisha Jackson, case manager, Triangle Insurance Co.

Exhibit 7-5. *Introduction letter to the client with traditional indemnity insurance*

attends physician appointments. Most contact with the treating physician is telephonic.

One other main difference between health insurance and workers' compensation involves out-of-pocket expenses. The client injured at work does not pay any deductible or copay. All medical expenses are paid at 100 percent from the first dollar. In contrast, the client with traditional indemnity insurance must reach an annual, predetermined deductible. In addition, the client is often responsible for 20 percent of approved medical costs up to a certain dollar amount. Thus the case manager needs to advise the client of anticipated expenses while coordinating the plan of care.

Upon receipt of the referral, the case manager contacts the insurance company case manager to review specific requests. After the introduction letter is sent to the client, the case manager contacts the client to arrange an appointment.

THE PROCESS

The case management practice guidelines, which were developed through a collaborative project between Aetna Health Plans and the Individual Case Management Association (ICMA) in 1996, list five stages within the case management process. Whereas the stages are the same as the nursing process in general, carrying out the process is unique to case management. The five stages are (1) assessment, (2) planning, (3) implementation, (4) evaluation, and (5) documentation.

Assessment

Before the assessment is begun, the case manager must inform the client about the case manager's role and the scope of case management activities. The patient must be aware that using case management is voluntary and that the case manager will share information with the payer.[5] The concept of "informed consent" applies to the case management process. The client will be asked to sign a consent for release of medical information, which should be explained to the client simply but completely.

The assessment stage involves information gathering. The sources of information and the assessment tool are discussed in depth in Chapter 4. The success of the case management process depends on a thorough, objective, and comprehensive assessment.

During the course of data collection, the case manager begins identifying the client's needs and any issues or barriers that may interfere with the provision of care and expected outcomes. Such barriers may include experimental or alternative treatment, lack of family members or significant others, living in rural or remote areas, or religious beliefs that prohibit certain medical procedures.[6]

Planning

After all the data are collected and analyzed, the case manager, in collaboration with all providers and the client, develops an individualized case management plan. A comprehensive plan includes activities necessary to meet the client's needs across the continuum of the health care delivery system and throughout the entire episode of illness or injury. The plan should also include recommendations for alternative care and the costs of treatment.[7]

Recommended actions will depend upon the benefit package, state mandates (when workers' compensation is involved), and the client's individual decisions regarding his or her health care. To clearly understand the client's wishes, the case manager should discuss advance directives with the client, family members, and the physician before recommending any course of action. Extracontractual benefits may be considered after exhausting all approaches within the benefit package. It is often more cost-effective to design a plan extracontractually rather than to rigidly adhere to the plan.

Long- and short-term goals are developed during the planning stage of the case management process.[8] Goals should be appropriate, realistic, and measurable.

Implementation

Based on the case management plan, the case manager facilitates the coordination of appropriate, high-quality, cost-effective and time-effective care as the client moves through the health care delivery system. However, prior to implementation, the case manager contacts the payer to discuss the recommended actions. The case manager must realize that "no plan will be instituted until the case manager has obtained acceptance and agreement of all parties, i.e., patient/member and family, payer and physician/providers."[9]

Upon receiving approval to proceed, the case manager uses negotiation, communication, and collaboration to coordinate services with various providers. Through careful planning, knowledge of resources and appropriate coordination, duplication of services is avoided, fragmentation is decreased, and the client receives appropriate, cost-effective care.

Evaluation

After the case management plan has been instituted, the case manager must evaluate its effectiveness. The questions that the case manager must answer include (1) Is the plan working? (2) Is the patient satisfied? (3) Is the payer satisfied? (4) Is the patient compliant? (5) Are all the client's needs being met? and (6) Is the plan cost-effective?[10]

Often, the case management plan needs revision. The plan may not be effective, the client may not be satisfied and/or the client's status may change. Problem identification, resolution, evaluation, and reevaluation is continuous throughout the case management process. During the evaluation and reevaluation stages the case manager is an active participant. Case managers do not "monitor" the client's status, which implies passivity. The case manager should remain actively involved in the continuous and cyclical nature of the case management process.

Documentation

As with all areas of health care, documentation is essential. The method of documentation used by the external case manager is in written reports. Regardless of the format, "documentation must be objective, factual, clear and concise."[11] Since the report is often read by people who are not health professionals, medical terminology should be avoided or explained.

Documentation is necessary throughout each stage of the case management process. Goals and expected outcomes must be included. Each report should include what the case manager did, the rationale behind the actions, and the outcomes derived from the activity.

Reports should also include the cost of care coordinated by the case manager, projected costs, and the savings generated through the case management process. The case manager documents both hard and soft savings.

Hard savings are the actual cost of care that has been avoided through case management. For example, a case manager is working with a client who is going to be transferred to a subacute facility. The case manager contacts the facility to determine the cost, which is quoted as $800/day. Through negotiating with the subacute facility, the rate is decreased to $550/day. The case manager documents hard savings of $250/day for each day of the client's stay in the subacute facility.

Soft savings are more difficult to measure but are a direct result of effective case management. Soft savings reflect the avoidance of potential charges, rather than actual costs. As an example, a case manager may be working with a client diagnosed with asthma. This client has a history of hospitalizations every 3 months due to exacerbation of his asthma. The average length of stay has been 3 days, at a total cost to the carrier of $3,000. The case manager determines that the client does not have a thorough understanding of what triggers an attack, nor does the client use the inhaler properly. By teaching the client how to use the inhaler appropriately and to avoid certain triggers, the client remains out of the hospital for the following 6 months. The case manager would document the soft savings as $3,000 for 3 days in the hospital that were avoided as a direct result of case management. (See Appendix I for examples of reports and cost savings.)

Case management reports are often the only documentation that clearly and concisely outline the chronological events, care, and outcomes for a client, across the continuum and through the entire episode of illness or injury. The report reflects collaborative efforts and includes recommendations made from all members of the health care team.

Chapter
Highlights

* The case management process closely parallels the nursing process in general; however, case management is more global and long-term
* Although a universal model of the case management process does not yet exist, there have been recent efforts to develop such a model that is both comprehensive and future-oriented.
* The case management process begins with receipt of a referral. The focus of the case management process will vary depending on the payer source (workers' compensation versus traditional indemnity health insurance)
* The case manager working with clients injured at work is bound by specific state guidelines and legislation.
* The case manager working with clients with traditional indemnity health insurance is able to be more creative in developing a case management plan.
* The actual case management process includes five stages. These five stages are (1) assessment, (2) planning, (3) implementation, (4) evaluation, and (5) documentation.
* Each stage of the process depends upon successful and comprehensive completion of the previous stage. The process is cyclical in nature and requires ongoing revision and reevaluation. Documentation is carried out through each stage of the process.
* Documentation of both hard and soft savings is an essential part of the case management process.

*   The goal of the case management process is to achieve high-quality, cost-effective, and time-effective coordination of care across the continuum and through the entire episode of injury or illness.

1. Hoeman, S. (1996). Case management. *Rehabilitation nursing: process and application.* (2d ed.). St. Louis, MO: Mosby. p. 102.
2. Ibid.
3. Newell, M. (1996). *Using nursing case management to improve health outcomes.* Gaithersburg, MD: Aspen. p. 20.
4. Newell, M. (1996). *Using nursing case management to improve health outcomes.* Gaithersburg, MD: Aspen. p. 21.
5. St. Coeur, M. (1996). *Case management practice guidelines.* St. Louis, MO: Mosby. p. 3.
6. Ibid., p. 4.
7. Hoeman, Case management. p. 103.
8. St. Coeur, *Case management practice guidelines.* p. 5.
9. Ibid.
10. Ibid., p. 6.
11. Ibid., p. 7.

CHAPTER

Measuring Quality ⟨ 8 ⟩
and Case
Management

Nursing case management has been adopted across the continuum of health care delivery settings to provide a more effective care mechanism to achieve optimum client outcomes. But does it really work? As with all aspects of health care delivery, there must be some means in place to evaluate how well the process is working. For case management, questions such as these should be addressed: Were the services coordinated effectively? Were the appropriate services obtained? What was the quality of the services? Have the specific needs of the client been met? Was in fact the entire process cost-effective? This chapter will briefly review the traditional methods used to assess the quality of health care and then focus on the most current model, continuous quality improvement (CQI).

Upon completion of this chapter, you will be able to answer the following questions:

1. How was traditional quality assurance limited in creating positive change in health care delivery?
2. What factors promoted the development of CQI in health care delivery?
3. How have principles of total quality management (TQM) been integrated into health care evaluation?

4. How do case managers apply measurement of variance as a component of CQI efforts?
5. What opportunities exist for case managers to contribute to CQI efforts in their work environment?

TRADITIONAL QUALITY ASSURANCE (QA)

The concept of monitoring and evaluating the quality of health care is relatively new to health care delivery. Most nurses and health care providers tend to believe they can intuitively identify good versus bad practice and determine when the patient outcomes are satisfactory. Inherent in this assumption is the notion that all providers are equally knowledgeable and competent and working to meet the highest standard of care. In the real world, however, this is not the case. *Quality assurance* evolved to provide a "system of procedures used to evaluate nursing care and to give feedback to the providers of this service in order to improve it."[1]

Early evaluations of system quality were driven by requirements of Medicare and Medicaid statutes, increasing concern of state licensing agencies, provider agencies themselves, and the Joint Commission on Accreditation of Healthcare Organizations (JCAHO). Quality assurance focused on improving care only after problems were identified. Generally, an individual or team evaluated selected aspects of care directed by the organization. The team collected and organized data that would monitor the chosen aspects of care. Each aspect of care could be assessed by predetermined clinical indicators. Since some variation in care and outcome were expected, thresholds were established (a *threshold* could be a level, pattern, or trend) that when reached would trigger the initiation of the evaluation process. The result of the evaluation process included taking action to improve care, correct identified problems, document improvement in care, and communicate findings to appropriate people and departments in the system. The overall concern of traditional quality assurance monitoring was to determine whether the services provided had met the designated standards. This ensured that all professional practice was at least satisfactory in terms of standards but did little to consider how the overall system might be improved.

Quality assurance monitoring was accomplished from two different time perspectives. *Concurrent review* entailed systematically evaluating current performance. *Retrospective review* focused on past performance. Regardless of the time perspective, the primary data collection procedure was the chart audit. The chart audit involved determining appropriateness of diagnostic tests and treatments as well as overall utilization of resources.

As a first step toward considering the outcomes of health care, quality assurance programs have some utility. The QA model focuses on four steps: (1) monitor for quality, (2) identify a problem, (3) take corrective action, and (4) remonitor to see if the problem is resolved. Quality is measured from the perspective of the number of errors made or accidents occurring. As a result, "bad apples" (e.g., clinicians making medication errors, using poor judgment) can be pinpointed and corrective action can be taken.

However, one limitation of this strategy is that any problems discovered often appear to be the fault of an individual or small group. Because of its focus on single events, the model of traditional quality assurance does not really provide an opportunity to explore all the factors present that can contribute to problem areas. For example, often the structure of the system or processes crossing system boundaries lead to problems. In addition, the mind-set underpinning quality assurance lacks comprehensive vision—little attention is paid to the system as a whole, how to enhance system performance, or how to deliver a higher-quality or more desirable product. Because of its restricted focus and lack of multidisciplinary involvement, traditional quality assurance can induce a degree of inertia into the system, leaving limited ability to anticipate or respond to external forces that indicate a need for change. Because of the changes experienced by the health care industry through the 1980s and as attention focused increasingly on cost and product, a different perspective for evaluation was needed.

TOTAL QUALITY MANAGEMENT

Providers of health care are now fiercely competing, driven by the need to produce higher-quality care at lower costs. Because there is a surplus of providers (this includes physicians, hospitals, clinical laboratories and diagnostic services, equipment vendors, and the like), only those who are efficient and effective obtain a market share of the "customers" (health care consumers). Managed care insurance companies negotiate contracts with the most cost-effective providers. Newer types of hybrid insurance coverage offered by consortia of providers which share financial risk can only survive if the care delivered is both effective in outcomes and efficient in cost.

Legal and regulatory changes now promote reconsideration of how health care systems operate and measure quality. In several malpractice suits against physicians, not only were the physicians found guilty but also the hospitals in which they were practicing. The courts raised issues that suggest that the hospital has a responsibility to monitor and ensure the quality of the system of care.

In a similar vein, JCAHO has established an agenda for change in which it calls for "a new, more positive approach called continuous quality improvement . . . adapting the philosophy and tools that industries have used to effectively improve the levels of quality in their products and services."[2]

The concept of increasing quality to obtain competitive advantage developed as an industrial model to enhance manufacturing processes. Working with Japanese manufacturers following World War II, W. Edwards Deming and Joseph Juran proposed a production model that would "create a process for improving the quality of products and services produced by an organization."[3] Deming envisioned that *total quality management* (TQM) would provide a strategy for a "structured, systematic process for creating organization-wide participation in planning and implementing continuous improvements in quality. TQM is a means to an end with the end being the long-term success of an organization."[4]

In essence, Deming and Juran believed that the key to successful quality management was developing an organizational culture based on participative systems focused on the search for ways to improve quality. All employees become contributing team members "emphasizing interconnectedness, customer service, system improvement, and team performance to achieve the goal of meeting or exceeding customer needs and expectations."[5] The underlying philosophy of the organization was critical, since a serious commitment from top management was essential to remove barriers within the organization that would in any way diminish the collaborative effort of all workers. Deming's model integrates 14 guidelines for quality improvement that, working in unison, will accomplish transformation of any business. The 14 points focus on three concepts: leadership and team building, empowering the worker, and changing the philosophy of the organization. Deming asserts that it is critical for businesses to establish long-term views regarding employees, products, supplier relationships, and profitability.[6]

Quality is defined by two factors: meeting or exceeding the customer's expectations (*customer satisfaction*) and achieving this goal at a reasonable price (*salability*). Within the TQM model, if all system efforts are dedicated to meeting customer expectations at a competitive price, success is likely to occur.

APPLYING TQM TO HEALTH CARE— CONTINUOUS QUALITY IMPROVEMENT

Total quality management has had impressive effects on many industries. However, in health care, no tangible "product" is produced. Rather, the only product is really a service that "cannot be disassociated from the production process or person providing the service."[7] And there is no way to store or inventory a service for later demand, as you would a product or type of merchandise. Thus, there is always a potential for problems created by waiting times and coordination between caregivers, since not all client needs can be predicted. Anyone with personal experience in the delivery of health care will recognize how true this is.

Because we are focusing on a service, it is difficult to achieve consensus for a definition of *quality*. The current trend is to include objective elements such as health status (an outcome) and subjective elements such as client satisfaction. Another complicating factor when defining quality is that neither clients nor providers are homogeneous. Clients have individual needs, beliefs, preferences, and lifestyles. Providers strive to individualize care by balancing their own treatment preferences (which often relate to where and how they were educated or to personal beliefs regarding efficacy) with what they believe will be most acceptable to the particular client. In essence, there are relatively few "norms" regarding treatment protocols for most health problems, leaving substantial latitude in choice of treatment to the individual physician and client.

Despite these acknowledged limitations, continuous quality improvement does provide a systematic and systemic approach to improving clinical outcomes and agency performance. CQI achieves this by: (1) identifying what customers need and want, (2) exploring the processes in use to deliver services using a multidisciplinary team, and (3) analyzing how processes can be modified to reduce variation and improve customer satisfaction. CQI supports our efforts to watch for opportunities to make the system better.

The Customer Focus

Focus on the customer is a cornerstone of CQI. From the perspective of a health care delivery system, there are both internal and external customers. *Internal customers* include any employee or process that relies on input from another part of the system to carry out the assigned responsibilities. For example, an important aspect of the nurse's role is administration of medication as ordered. To implement this role effectively and efficiently, many components of the health care system must interact: The physician writes the order; a designated employee transcribes the order; the order is communicated to the pharmacy through some predetermined process; the pharmacy reviews the order for appropriateness and then fills the order by dispensing the medication (which has been previously supplied by an outside vendor); the medication must be physically delivered to the nursing unit; it must then be stored; the nurse administers the medication at the proper time, using appropriate supplies and/or materials for administration that must be available; the nurse records the administration and assesses the client for the effects of the medication; the nurse communicates with the physician regarding the effect of the medication.

In the above scenario, multiple employees and departments are involved in the completion of a single component of client care—administration of medication. All these employees and processes are considered internal customers.

Numerous external customers must also be considered. The client seeking health care service is the primary external customer. However, the providers of health care who are not system employees (for example, private or attending physicians) are also external customers as they have the option to "take their business elsewhere." Likewise, insurance companies have become major customers of health care agencies. Insurance companies enter into contracts with those selected agencies that they expect will provide the most cost-effective quality care. Given the oversupply of most types of providers and agencies, the insurance companies have substantial economic power as customers. Using CQI, every characteristic of services provided and processes used with which a customer might be concerned is explored.

Understanding the Customer

We must always look for opportunities to become more involved with our customers. By doing this, we develop greater awareness of who our customers are, their preferences, and concepts of how services should be provided; we also establish open lines of communication. Several strategies are used to gather information from and about our customers. The two most popular techniques are focus groups and written surveys.

A *focus group* is a qualitative research strategy that uses group discussion to explore a set of predetermined questions. Generally, 6 to 10 people with knowledge of the area under investigation are invited to participate in a 45- to 60-minute discussion led by a trained facilitator. Often the sessions are tape-recorded so all information is captured.

Let's say that a hospital is interested in determining what types of additional services it might plan to develop for the future. One mechanism for gathering information in this area would be to conduct focus groups with community leaders, residents, and health care providers to explore their views on this question.

Alternatively, an independent case manager might be interested in evaluating customer satisfaction of clients who have already received case management services. Exhibit 8-1 is an example of a typical survey that could be used for this purpose.

Measuring Quality

Quality improvement strives to ensure that "every aspect of a job is consistently done right the first time."[8] If this occurs, there would be minimal variation in both the processes of delivering care and in the outcomes of such care. In the real world, it is unreasonable to expect this degree of perfection. Health care delivery requires the interaction of professional and nonprofessional caregivers and employees, numerous departments that provide different services, external vendors of supplies and equipment, and a client who is unique in "being" and in response to treatment modalities. Thus, the process of care, "a set of causes and conditions that repeatedly come together to transform inputs into outcomes,"[9] normally creates some variation. Variation is generally one of two types; *common variation*, which is an inherent element within the system or process, and *special variation*, which is caused by a transient or unique event. Since common variation is the direct result of the processes

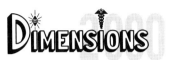

in Managed Care

Sandy Mandell, MA, CRRN, CIRS, CCM
DIRECTOR
201-882-8512

NAME:(optional) _____ DATE: _____

Your Case Manager: _____

　　To achieve continuing quality improvement, your input and comments are important. Our goal is to provide high-quality service, with an emphasis on open communication. We would appreciate if you would complete this questionnaire and return it in the enclosed stamped, self-addressed envelope. Please feel free to add as many comments or suggestions as you like. If you need additional space, use the back of this sheet.

　　Please be assured that this survey does not affect your benefits in any way. We are seeking your honest opinion and suggestions, so that we can continue to fulfill your health care needs in the most appropriate and caring manner.

　　Call me at anytime (800-555-5555) to discuss any case management issues.

PLEASE READ THE STATEMENT AND THEN CHECK THE BOX WHICH YOU BELIEVE BEST FITS

	Strongly Agree	Usually Agree	Sometimes Agree	Never Agree
1. My case manager returns my calls promptly.	☐	☐	☐	☐
2. Case management has improved the quality of my care.	☐	☐	☐	☐
3. My case manager interprets "medical words" so I can better understand my diagnosis and treatment.	☐	☐	☐	☐

Exhibit 8-1.　*Client satisfaction survey*

	Strongly Agree	Usually Agree	Sometimes Agree	Never Agree
4. My case manager really cares about my well-being.	☐	☐	☐	☐
5. My case manager only cares about saving money	☐	☐	☐	☐
6. Case management has cut out a lot of "red tape."	☐	☐	☐	☐
7. My case manager knows about community resources for those things that are not covered in my policy.	☐	☐	☐	☐
8. I was originally doubtful about case management and felt that this was only another way to cut my benefits.	☐	☐	☐	☐
9. My case manager directs my care without discussing it with me first.	☐	☐	☐	☐
10. When I need to talk, I know I can call my case manager.	☐	☐	☐	☐

PLEASE COMPLETE THE FOLLOWING SENTENCES:

1. The thing I like most about case management is _____

_____

2. The thing I dislike most about case management is

_____

ADDITIONAL COMMENTS OR SUGGESTIONS (IF YOU NEED MORE SPACE, USE THE BACK OF THIS SHEET).

_____

_____

_____

involved, this type of variation can be reduced only by changing the process. Alternatively, special variation is caused by factors outside of the process and can therefore be reduced only by eliminating the cause. Within the health care environment, a focus on controlling or eliminating common variation will yield the greatest sustained improvement in the efficiency of operation.

Refer to the previous scenario on medication administration, since it can exemplify common and special variation. Using the assessment data from routine auditing procedures, medication error reports, and anecdotal reports from nursing staff as well as from patient surveys, we know that 20 percent of the medications ordered are not administered within the specified time frames. This is a serious concern because it can lead to decreased patient satisfaction, delay in carrying out other diagnostic and treatment protocols, and even slower patient recovery. Further analysis of the data using statistical tools such as flowcharts and histograms helps answer the following questions:

- What might be the cause(s) of the problem and the associated effects of the causes?
- How might relationships among time of day, day of week, personnel assigned, nursing unit, types of patients, and the administration of medication affect outcomes?
- Are there factors, previously unrecognized, that are contributing to difficulties in administration of medication on time?

Let's say that in 80 percent of the cases when the medication was not administered on time, the cause was found to be that the medication was not yet available on the nursing unit. Further analysis determines that this occurs most frequently within the first 12 hours after patient admission. This is a form of common variation and can be directly related to the existing procedures in use regarding medication orders, transcription, and processing to the point of getting the medication stock to the unit for administration. Although efforts to amend procedures must be vigorous and require collaboration of the several disciplines involved in the problematic work process, once a new process is undertaken, it is possible virtually to eliminate this common variation as a source of difficulty.

Documenting Variation

Understanding variation is enhanced by the use of critical pathways. A *critical pathway* is a multidisciplinary, comprehensive guide that describes the course of care for a client with a specific diagnosis according to DRG. The pathway lists the key events, potential problems, specific interventions, and expected outcomes to be achieved for each patient with a given diagnosis. These elements are projected along a timeline which designates exactly when interventions are to occur. In essence, the critical pathway establishes the ideal diagnostic and treatment plan for a diagnosis by laying out all processes of care the client requires. This type of standardization is a critical component of CQI efforts.

Variance occurs any time the patient does not progress as outlined in the critical pathway and usually indicates a lag in moving toward anticipated outcomes. Variance can be *operational*: (1) the result of problems related to the system (e.g., an MRI is ordered but the equipment is being serviced, resulting in a delay of 8 hours for the diagnostic test) or related to the health care provider (e.g., the neuroradiologist who must interpret the MRI is not available), or (2) *patient related* (e.g., the patient is experiencing severe anxiety about having the MRI and refuses to have the test at this time). Documentation of all variances is an ongoing, daily process using formats specific to the institution. This type of data collection allows for analysis of every failure of a client to reach expected outcomes. When variances are created by health care provider behaviors, the documentation does not go in the patient's medical record. For medicolegal reasons, such variances are usually recorded in "unusual occurrence reports" or "incident reports." Variances due to system factors are also generally recorded on forms other than the patient's medical record.

Patient-related variance occurs for many reasons. Sometimes a patient may refuse a test or treatment, may have an unpredicted response to treatment, or may have an alteration in function such as a spike in temperature. Often a patient-related variance provides the first indication that the patient's condition is deteriorating. Careful attention to details can help determine the cause of a variance. For example, consider an 80-year-old client who is recovering from an open reduction and internal fixation of a fractured hip. On the first postoperative day, the client is to begin physical therapy for leg exercises. The nurse notes at 8 p.m. that exercises were not carried out. Why? Was the omission system-related? Was it provider-related? Or was it patient-related? In this case it was due to several patient factors. The patient was agitated and angry because his daughter had just told him that he would not be able to return to live with her after discharge. The patient had slept poorly the night before because of pain. The current pain medication was not adequate to relieve symptoms, and the patient had frequently requested additional medication. Finally, the patient did not speak English and relied heavily on his daughter to serve as a translator. Bottom line, the patient refused to participate in exercises when the physical therapist came to see him. In this example, a single variance documenting noncompliance with the physical therapy treatment protocol provided the initial indication that multiple client and family needs had to be addressed. In a case like this, the variance documentation relating specifically to the patient and family would be made in the progress notes component of the patient's medical record.

When variances are believed to be the result of complex causes, the best course of action is to hold a multidisciplinary case consultation. These short meetings (usually requiring 15 to 20 minutes) allow for input from all providers involved in the patient's care. The discussion will focus on determining whether the critical pathway is realistic for this patient as well as whether the variance problem can be resolved. Often, the initial assessment of the patient's abilities may be found to have been in error, and therefore the standardized critical pathway really cannot work for the particular person. Alternatively, there may be true deterioration in the patient's condition, so that anticipated outcomes, time frames, and interventions have to be reconsidered and redefined.

In the example of the client with a hip fracture, a case consultation was held to explore sources of variance. The actual discussion required only 11 minutes and included input from the nurse, physical therapist, social worker, and surgeon. It was determined that the critical pathway was appropriate for the patient, but a few modifications would be necessary. The medication regimen was altered, the social worker scheduled a conference with the family on that day, and a worker in a nearby department was contacted to serve as interpreter as needed. For a rather modest investment of time as a resource, the case conference was invaluable not only in identifying the source of the difficulty but also in resolving it.

THE CASE MANAGER'S ROLE IN CQI

Case managers have a significant role in the CQI efforts of any health care system. Since the essence of case management is its focus on expediting all processes involved in delivering care to effect a speedy client recovery, achievement of maximum level of wellness, and timely return to work, the case manager is well attuned to a *customer focus*. Case managers in any setting, whether or not involved in the direct delivery of nursing care, are always searching for ways to refine care delivery to achieve outcomes more economically. By virtue of their experience and education, case managers have the mind-set that a foundation of better health care rests on improved design of services and reduction of variation in processes.

In inpatient settings, case managers participate as members of multidisciplinary teams to improve processes that can really make a difference in patient care. They are involved in identifying the *priority areas* worth monitoring (as part of the CQI program), since it just is not possible or realistic to change everything in a system. Case managers also collect data for analysis. Do note that, depending on the scope of the process being assessed as well as the type of data collected, collaboration with a statistician may be required.

Outside the acute care or similar facility, external case managers are involved in CQI primarily when working independently at the behest of a client. In this case, a major focus is on assessing exactly what the customer wants and then developing a plan to deliver the care and evaluate outcomes as well as customer satisfaction. If the customer is an insurance carrier, the carrier probably wants a satisfied patient whose health care needs have been met at the lowest possible cost to the insurance company. At times, the external case manager can find it extremely difficult to mediate the interests of the two clients—the insurance carrier who wishes to save dollars and the patient who wants as much care and service as possible, which entails the spending of dollars.

THE FUTURE OF CQI

Depending on where you live and work, you will find that there are immense differences in the degree to which health care facilities are embracing the concept of CQI. In some areas of the country, traditional quality assurance programs prevail, and nurses as well as other team members are just now beginning to explore the use of the CQI model. In other areas, sophisticated CQI programs are up and running, with complex data collection being carried out by integrated computer systems in the facility. In the latter case, the more advanced health care agencies are likely to be using critical paths for numerous DRGs and are probably *benchmarking* (measuring key work processes in the facility and comparing the results with those of the best performers, usually outside the facility) against comparable facilities in the area, state, or even nation.

Regardless of the employment setting for the case manager, involvement in continuous quality improvement activities will certainly be a component of our role. Clearly, this element of health care delivery will continue to expand as market forces drive systems to be more competitive, economical, and sensitive to the varied interests and needs of both internal and external customers.

Chapter
Highlights

* Traditional quality assurance monitors care and operations of a system to maintain minimum performance standards.

* The restricted focus of quality assurance and increasing demands of regulatory bodies supported the evolution of quality assurance into continuous quality improvement.
* Continuous quality improvement in the health care industry has drawn heavily on the models of Deming and Juran which had been developed for manufacturing industries.
* Many terms are applied to current initiatives in quality management—*continuous quality improvement* and *total quality management* are the most common.
* Continuous quality improvement strives to improve clinical outcomes and agency performance by focusing on customer needs and desires and on how the processes of care delivery can be improved.
* The case manager's role in continuous quality improvement is primarily to explore sources of and solutions to variance.

References

1. Tappen, R. (1995). *Nursing leadership and management: concepts and practice* (3d ed.). Philadelphia, Pa: F.A. Davis. p. 461.
2. Joint Commission on Accreditation of Healthcare Organizations. (1991). *Transitions: from QA to CQI.* Oakbrook Terrace, IL. p. 3.
3. Whetsell, G. (1991). Total quality management. *Topics in health care financing.* 18(2), 12–20.
4. Ibid.
5. Langlais, R. (1996, Jan-Feb). Recognizing organizational impediments to the total quality management process. *Best Practices and Benchmarking in Healthcare.* (1)1, 16.
6. Dienemann, J. (1992). *C.Q.I. Continuous quality improvement in nursing.* Washington, DC: American Nurses Publishing. p. 27.
7. Ibid., p. 20.
8. Ibid., p. 34.
9. Moen, R., & Nolan, T. (1987). Process improvement. *Quality Progress.* 4, 62–68.

Life Care Planning 9

The concept of life care planning (LCP) as developed by Paul Deutsch and Frederick Raffa in 1981 is a comprehensive, dynamic, and interdisciplinary approach to estimating the long- and short-term needs of the catastrophically injured person. Those needs are then translated into cost over the projected lifetime of the injured person.

Life care plans are used by insurance companies to set aside sufficient dollar "reserves" to cover the medical and general care expenses for a catastrophically injured person. This can often amount to several million dollars over the course of a person's remaining lifetime. Attorneys also use life care plans to help settle negligence or malpractice suits brought by severely disabled clients.

As with effective case management, life care plans call for an interdisciplinary effort. Collaboration with all team members is essential to produce an accurate and comprehensive estimate of needs and associated costs. The life care plan considers all medical/surgical, nursing, therapeutic, transportation, psychological, and vocational needs as well as equipment, supplies, and home modifications required. Such plans are not generic to a given diagnosis; rather, they reflect the individual needs of a specific person in a specific situation. In essence, a life care plan is the sum of all current and future needs of a catastrophically injured client throughout the projected life span.

complex, high-tech piece of equipment, such as an environmental control unit, which can open doors, turn lights on and off, answer phones, control temperature, start and stop computers, and so on through voice activation.

7. *Orthotics and prosthetics.* Amputees will need prostheses, which need replacement and ongoing maintenance. When the injured client is a child, the prosthesis will need replacement during growth stages. Brain or spinal cord-injured people may require braces or ankle and/or foot orthoses, which can be quite expensive when custom-designed.

8. *Home furnishings and accessories.* This area includes furniture and related accessories.

9. *Drug and supply needs.* This section includes all prescription and nonprescription medications and supplies. The most common supplies include catheters, leg bags, and bowel and bladder program supplies. For the ventilator-dependent client, additional items would include all tracheostomy supplies.

10. *Home care or facility care.* Although most people would choose to live in their home environment, this choice may be inappropriate or not feasible. For the client who is in a persistent vegetative state, quality care in a long-term care facility may be the best alternative for the family. The level of care and the age of the client may also influence the decision between home or facility. For example, an injured child may remain at home until the parents, or other caregivers, become too elderly to care for the adult dependent. A life care plan for this person would include home care needs until a certain age. Beyond that age the cost of a long-term care facility would be incorporated into the plan.

11. *Future medical care–routine.* This area includes all routine medical evaluations, lab work, and x-rays. Depending on the level and nature of the injury, the evaluations can range from an annual physical exam to complex evaluations which include dental care, physiatry, urology, neurology, and others.

12. *Transportation.* Clients' transportation needs vary widely. Some clients may need only minor adaptations such as hand controls to make the currently owned vehicle usable in light of the disability. Other clients may need a custom-designed van with a wheelchair lift

and possibly a raised roof. The cost of registration is usually higher for a customized van than it is for a simple automobile. Therefore, the cost of annual registration is included in the life care plan.

13. *Recreation and leisure.* This section includes adaptive games and/or specialized equipment that the client will need to remain as active and independent as possible. Specialty wheelchairs for the wheelchair athlete would be included in this section.

14. *Architectural renovations.* If the client chooses to remain at home, costly home modifications may be necessary. The most common renovations include ramps, stair glides, widening of doors and hallways, enlargement of the bathroom, modified bathroom equipment, modifying the kitchen, and changing floor coverings.

15. *Potential complications.* At best, potential complications are difficult to predict. The client with a spinal cord injury may be very prone to skin breakdown. However with appropriate care, this complication can be avoided. The client with a brain injury has a high probability of falling due to loss of balance or poor judgment. Again, appropriate coordination of care can minimize this potential for injury.

Although many life care plans include the cost of potential complications, the Deutsch model lists the complications stating "for information only." Deutsch believes that it is important for people to realize that potential exists for various complications; however, with appropriate planning many of these complications can be avoided.

16. *Future medical care/surgical intervention or aggressive treatment.* Depending on the injury, certain surgical procedures may be necessary over a set time. For example, the client who has sustained severe burns will need multiple plastic and orthopedic surgeries. For a comprehensive life care plan, the case manager needs to assess the cost of the surgery and the projected length of hospital stay. Recuperative costs, such as temporary nursing care or physical therapy following surgery, must also be included.

17. *Orthopedic and other equipment needs.* Equipment needs vary with the type and level of injury. Common medical equipment (DME) includes hospital bed, commode, and bath and shower equipment. When working with a client who is ventilator-dependent, the equipment needs are obviously greater. The case manager

must include the cost of maintenance or service contracts for items that will be purchased (as opposed to rented). The case manager must also include the cost of a backup ventilator and a compressor for emergency use during electrical failure.

18. *Vocational and educational plan.* This section is often completed by a vocational counselor. The information documented in this area includes the cost of job coaching, vocational counseling, tuition fees, books and supplies and/or specialized educational programs.[3]

CASE STUDY

The following case study of an uncomplicated client situation is an abbreviated form of an actual life care plan report using the Deutsch format (from *A Guide to Rehabilitation*, Paul M. Deutsch, Ph.D. & Horace Sawyer, Ed.D., Matthew Bender, New York). This particular client would require only a minimum amount of services. In practice, you will find that clients needing life care plans have been severely injured and their independence as well as their cognitive and/or physiologic functions have been severely compromised.

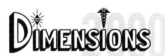

in Managed Care
LIFE CARE PLAN

Client: Mr. Quinn
Social Security Number: 111-11-1111   Date of birth: January 5, 19XX
Date of evaluation: February 1, 19XX
Date of report: March 15, 19XX

In preparing this life care plan the following medical records were reviewed:

- Mercy Hospital chart from November 3, 19XX through December 15, 19XX
- Well Spring Rehabilitation Center chart from December 15, 19XX through February 15, 19XX

- Outpatient physical and occupational therapists' evaluation reports and progress notes from February 17, 19XX through March 1, 19XX
- Hospital admission and discharge medical records dated: April 5–8, 19XX; November 3–5, 19XX; March 20–30, 19XX; January 10–13, 19XX; and October 17–20, 19XX
- Telephone interviews with Dr. Abdul (physiatrist), Dr. Boyle (psychologist), and Dr. Chatsworth (urologist)
- Personal interview with the client, his wife, and his mother

I. Introduction

Mr. Quinn is a 30-year-old male diagnosed with T-3 paraplegia secondary to a motor vehicle accident which occurred on November 3, 19XX.

The purpose of this evaluation was to assess the extent to which this individual has incurred disabilities secondary to his injury. The manner in which these disabilities impede his future vocational development and the extent to which they interfere with his ability to demonstrate independent living skills or handle activities of daily living will be explored in the conclusions and appendixes attached to this report.

In addition to the client, his wife and mother were present throughout the interview.

Mr. Quinn gives a history of a head-on collision that occurred on November 3, 19XX. He has no memory of the details of the accident. His first memory following the accident is at the hospital. Mrs. Quinn stated that her husband was airlifted to Mercy Hospital, where he remained an inpatient for 6 weeks. During the course of hospitalization he underwent T-1 through T-6 fusion with insertion of rod and screws. In addition, he required plastic surgery for lacerations on the face and left forearm. Complications during hospitalization included an infected sacral decubitus. At discharge he was transferred to Well Spring Rehabilitation Center where he remained for 2 months. Following discharge from rehabilitation, Mr. Quinn continued with outpatient physical and occupational therapy for approximately one year.

When Mr. Quinn was discharged home he was independent with wheelchair mobility. He required minimal to moderate assistance in most activities of daily living; however, with adaptive devices and continued therapy his independence continued to increase.

Mr. Quinn stated that between April 19XX and the present he has been hospitalized five times for treatment of kidney stones, recurrent bladder infections, and a flap graft to the sacrum.

Mr. Quinn lives with his wife in a one-story ranch-style home. A ramp has been installed for entry; however, much of the interior remains only partially accessible. Mr. Quinn cannot maneuver in the bathroom without assistance and is unable to use many of the appliances in the kitchen.

Mrs. Quinn is employed full-time as a computer programmer approximately 45 minutes from the home. Mr. Quinn's mother visits frequently to assist with his care. Mr. Quinn does not have any siblings. His father was diagnosed with lung cancer 10 years ago and has been deceased for 8 years.

II. Chief complaints

Mr. Quinn is permanently disabled. Secondary to the paraplegia are problems with decubitus, urinary drainage, and a urethral tear. According to Dr. Chatsworth, Mr. Quinn's treating urologist, the recommended sphincterotomy cannot be performed until complicating urological problems are cleared.

Mr. Quinn's bowel program consists of digital stimulation and Theravac three times weekly. He states that he has been able to control his bowel movements with this program and has infrequent accidents.

Mr. Quinn's main complaint is pain. He states that he has constant pain and is often unable to sleep through the night.

III. Medical summary

Mr. Quinn states that he is 5'10" tall and weighs 200 lb. He states a 30-lb weight gain since the injury.

Mr. Quinn denies any serious injuries or illnesses prior to the accident. He denies smoking and states he is "a social drinker."

Mr. Quinn expressed anger and frustration concerning his disability. However, he stated that through psychological counseling he is beginning to accept his limitations and is anxious to begin setting vocational goals.

IV. Physical limitations

Mr. Quinn has total loss of movement and sensation below the T-3 level. He has no bowel or bladder control. He uses a wheelchair for mobility. Sitting balance is fair due to the level of injury.

Mr. Quinn has had recurrent decubiti and urological problems.

V. Current medical care

Mr. Quinn remains under the care of the following physicians:

Dr. Abdul, physiatrist
Dr. Boyle, psychologist
Dr. Chatsworth, urologist

Mr. Quinn takes the following medications:

Multivitamin: 1 daily
Theravac: 3 times weekly
Elavil: 50 mg at bedtime

VI. Educational/vocational history

At the time of injury Mr. Quinn was a second-year student at Midwestern University Law School. He graduated Southwest University as an undergraduate in 19XX with a BA degree in history. Mr. Quinn is anxious to return to school to complete his law education. Career goals include becoming an attorney specializing in negligence and malpractice cases.

Past vocational history includes odd jobs after school and on weekends. Mrs. Quinn has been the primary financial support system for herself and the client.

VII. Conclusion

Careful consideration has been given to all the medical, psychosocial, and rehabilitative information contained within this file and report. There is no question that Mr. Quinn is permanently disabled as a result of a motor vehicle accident.

As a result of Mr. Quinn's limitations, he needs assistance with household chores and home repairs, which he had been able to perform prior to the injury. As Mr. Quinn ages, his need for assistance with activities of daily living will increase.

Other essential needs that Mr. Quinn has as a result of the injury are as follows:

- Home modifications to maximize his independence
- A pain management program for chronic pain
- Psychological and sexual counseling
- Vocational and educational assistance
- Transportation and recreational equipment

All the other needs dictated by the onset of this disability are outlined
in the attached life care plan. Please note that all costs are based on 19XX
dollars.

AGE NOW: 30.3
REMAINING YEARS: 40.9
LIFE EXPECTANCY: 71.2

Life expectancy based on US Life Tables, Inc., in *Rules Governing the
Courts of the State of New Jersey,* 19XX.

(Following the narrative portion of the life care plan, 18 separate pages, one for each area previously discussed, are included as
appendixes. For our purpose only two areas are included as examples. The final page of the report is titled "Life care plan cost summary" and lists the total of each appendix, with a final grand total.)
See Tables 9-1 and 9-2.

Chapter
Highlights

* Life care plans are used by insurance companies and attorneys to determine the total needs of a client throughout the
  life span.
* Life care plans are the result of a multidisciplinary, collaborative effort.
* The process of life care planning is similar to the case management process. However, the life care plan does not include
  implementation, evaluation, or follow-up contact.
* The actual life care plan report includes a comprehensive narrative, followed by 18 areas that are outlined in terms of base
  cost, frequency of replacement, total number used within a
  given lifetime, and the total cost throughout the projected
  life span.

Table 9-1. Life care plan appendix: Wheelchair needs, accessories, and maintenance

Type	Age Purchased	Replacement Schedule	Purpose	Base Cost	Number Purchased	Total
Quickie II	30	3 years	Mobility	$2,800.00	14	$39,200.00
Stimulite cushion	30	Yearly	Prevent skin breakdown	300.00	41	12,300.00
Maintenance	30	Yearly	Maintenance, parts, labor	350.00	41	14,350.00
Wheelchair bag	30	Yearly	Carrying items	30.00	41	1,230.00
TOTAL:						$67,080.00

Table 9-2. Life care plan appendix: Transportation

Item	Age Purchased	Replacement Schedule	Base Cost	Number Purchased	Total
Van with hand controls and wheelchair lift	30	6 years	$33,000.00	6	$198,000.00
Insurance	30	Yearly	2,000.00 (avg)	41	82,000.00
Registration	30	Yearly	100.00	41	4,100.00
Maintenance	30	Yearly	300.00 (avg)	41	12,300.00
TOTAL:					$296,400.00

References

1. Deutsch, P., & Sawyer, H. (1990). *A guide to rehabilitation*. New York: Binder. p. 7b–19.
2. Weed, R., & Riddick, S. (1992, Jan.–Feb.–Mar.). Life care plans as a case management tool. *The Case Manager*. 3(1), 30.
3. Ibid., pp. 28–31.

CHAPTER

Legal and 10
Ethical Issues

Ethical issues, now more than ever, play crucial roles in health care and nursing in general and in case management specifically. Until recently, such issues as confidentiality, abortion, physician-assisted suicide, the patient's right to refuse treatment, or the parent's right to refuse to prolong the life of severely compromised premature infants and be indebted by huge medical bills were not discussed as openly as they can be today.

Advanced technology, combined with an unending quest to reduce the cost of health care, has placed the system in a position of finding solutions to enormous ethical dilemmas. An *ethical dilemma* exists when "there is a conflict between two or more equally desirable (or undesirable) courses of action in a given situation."[1] Should the client with advanced, metastasized cancer be given aggressive treatment when the physician can predict the treatment will fail? Should the client with newly diagnosed stage 1 cervical cancer have the right to refuse initial treatment, only to spend huge amounts of health care dollars when the disease progresses? Should the newborn diagnosed with anencephaly be given the same aggressive, life-saving treatment as another child with a brighter prognosis?

Many people believe that the moral answer to all these questions is yes. However, given the current limited resources and the economic inability in this country to treat all people for all things, what is ethical versus what is possible remains open to debate. It is difficult at best to sort out our own personal beliefs about morals and values when we consider how we feel about such ethical dilemmas. To be a health care practitioner means that we have to resolve what our own ethical limits are and how far we can stretch them to conform to an institution's rules or a patient's rights. In that way, the action decided upon as the "correct" alternative can be adhered to and constitutes ethical nursing practice.[2]

Legal issues of decision making come into play as well. Attorneys are increasingly naming case managers as defendants in negligence cases. Thus, the issues of confidentiality, privileged information, scope of practice, and accountability are being questioned in courts of law.

Ethical and legal issues are integral parts of the case manager's role. Each client brings unique problems and situations that must be dealt with in an ethical, legal fashion consistent with accepted standards of practice. This chapter will examine some of the ethical and legal issues that case managers currently face.

Upon completion of this chapter you will be able to answer the following questions:

1. What are the types of ethical dilemmas most commonly encountered by nurse case managers?
2. What resources are available to assist in resolving ethical dilemmas?
3. How do standards of care relate to defining appropriate care for the client?
4. What types of legal issues most commonly occur in case management?
5. How can the case manager decrease the potential for liability in practice?

ETHICAL PERSPECTIVES

Philosophers and ethicists have spent years developing perspectives for ethical decision making. When a conflict in values gives rise to an ethical dilemma, an appropriate course of action must be taken. The action is dependent upon the perspective, or value priority, taken. The literature outlines 12 traditionally accepted perspectives, many of which directly conflict. These perspectives include:

- *Altruism,* or love of others, is the guide in decision making. An altruistic person will do what is "best" even at the risk of personal harm.
- *Collectivism* and *utilitarianism* focus on the good of the whole over that of the individual.
- *Duty-based* decisions are based on responsibilities or are made within the boundaries of contractual agreements.
- *Stoicism* values personal courage more than interaction with others.
- *Ethics of caring* is the perspective of caring for others in need.
- *Rational paternalism* is the perspective of the decision maker who "knows" the best course of action for the recipient.
- The perspectives of *individualism, existentialism, libertarianism,* and *rights based ethics* focus on the individual's freedom of personal choice.
- *Egoism* bases decisions on what is best for the decision maker.[3]

ETHICAL DILEMMAS IN CASE MANAGEMENT

Nurses and case managers are frequently faced with ethical dilemmas. The actions taken to resolve these conflicts are often based on a combination of perspectives: those of the client, the case manager, and the other providers of care. At the root of many value conflicts is the philosophical rationale behind health care as a right or a privilege.

It has been traditionally accepted that all people have a basic *right to health.* This is not synonymous with a basic *right to health care.* A right to health is considered a negative right. "It is a right not to have one's health interfered with by others."[4] A right to health care is a positive right, or a right to receive goods and services which would improve or maintain a current health status.[5] An example of a right to health is the *Patient's Bill of Rights,* which was developed by the American Hospital Association in 1972. Today, some form of the Patient's Bill of Rights is found in all health care facilities and ensures that all patients will be given the basic human rights of respect, dignity, continuity of care, and information about their care (see Exhibit 10-1).

The distinction between the right to health and the right to health care has become blurred, resulting in philosophical and ethical debate among the members of the health care community as well as within the general public. As the cost of health care continues to increase, this ethical dilemma has become further entrenched in controversy.

Exhibit 10-1. Patient's Bill of Rights (Subacute Facility)

Medical Care

- To retain the services of a physician you choose, at your own expense or through a health care plan.
- To have a physician explain to you, in language that you understand, your complete medical condition, the treatment planned for your care, and the expected results of your treatment.
- To participate in planning your medical treatment and care.
- To refuse medication and treatment after you have been informed of the possible consequences of your decision. You may also refuse to participate in experimental research.

Freedom from abuse and restraints

- Freedom from physical and mental abuse.
- Freedom from chemical and physical restraints, unless they are authorized by a physician for a limited period of time to protect you or others from injury.

Finances

- To manage your own finances or to delegate the responsibility.
- To receive a written statement describing the services provided and the related charges.
- To receive a quarterly written account of all your funds and property that are deposited with the facility for your use and safekeeping.
- To have daily access during specified, reasonable hours to the money and property that you have deposited with the facility.

Physical and personal environment

- To live in safe, decent, and clean conditions.
- To be treated with courtesy, consideration, and respect.

Privacy and confidential treatment

- To have physical privacy. You must be allowed, for example, to maintain the privacy of your body during medical treatment and personal hygiene activities unless you need assistance for your own safety.
- To have reasonable opportunities for intimate physical and social interaction with other people.

Mail and telephones

- To receive and send your mail in unopened envelopes. You also have a right to request and receive assistance in reading and writing correspondence.
- To have private access to a telephone.

Visits and activities

- To meet with any visitors of your choice between 8 a.m. and 8 p.m. daily.
- To take part in the facility activities, and to meet with and participate in the activities of any social, religious, and community groups.
- To refuse to perform services for the facility.
- To request visits at any time by representatives of the religion of your choice.
- To participate in meals, recreation, and social activities without being subjected to discrimination based on your age, race, religion, sex, or nationality.

Discharge and transfers

- To discharge yourself by presenting a release signed by you, your next of kin, or your guardian.
- To be transferred or discharged only for one or more of the following reasons:

    In an emergency, with notification of your physician and your next of kin or guardian.

For medical reasons or to protect your welfare or the welfare of others.

For nonpayment of fees, in situations not prohibited by law.

- To receive notice at least 10 days in advance when the facility requests your transfer or discharge, except in an emergency.

Protection of your rights

- To be given a written statement of your rights as well as any additional regulations established by the facility involving your rights and responsibilities. Copies should also be given to your family and the staff.
- To retain and exercise all constitutional, civil, and legal rights to which you are entitled by law. The facility is required to encourage and help you to exercise these rights.

Complaints and questions

- You have the right to voice complaints without being threatened or punished. The facility is required to provide you and your next of kin or guardian with the names, addresses, and telephone numbers of the government agencies to which you can complain and ask questions. This information must also be posted in a conspicuous place near every public telephone and on all public bulletin boards in the facility.

Source: With permission from Lakeview Subacute Care Center, Wayne, NJ.

Rationing Health Care

The idea of rationing health care is distasteful to many people. However, the cost of health care has reached a level which this nation can no longer afford. Managed care has grown exponentially in the past 2 years as a cost-saving method of delivering health care. Stringent limitations continue to be placed on health benefits within both managed care settings and on traditional indemnity insurance policies. No longer can the injured or ill person receive any and all treatments that the physician or the patient deem appropriate.

Issues that are currently being debated include coverage for injuries sustained by a reckless, possibly illegal act by the victim; illness caused by noncompliance with medical treatment or long-term maintenance of a high-risk lifestyle; liver transplants on a known alcoholic; performing a mastectomy on a 90-year-old woman diagnosed with breast cancer; using aggressive, high-tech lifesaving treatment for a newborn with multiple anomalies and a poor prognosis for survival; or spending millions of limited health care dollars treating illegal aliens, or people who come to this country for the specific purpose of receiving medical care.

As health care resources in America continue to shrink, the debate over rationing continues to increase. Many people may feel completely opposed to limiting medical treatment under any circumstances. However, when resources are finite, and it is their child who is denied treatment due to lack of funding, their perspectives may be altered. Rationing health care is a ubiquitous ethical dilemma, without easy solutions.

Overinvolvement

All nurses, regardless of their role, will at some time in their careers face the ethical dilemma of overinvolvement. Case managers, who establish relationships beyond the limitations of "hands on" care, and who may continue to provide services for several years or more, have an increased risk of becoming emotionally "attached" to a client. Once the nurse becomes overinvolved, does she automatically lose her ability to look at the client objectively? Can the nurse separate her personal feelings from her professional responsibilities?

For example, a case manager has worked with a severely debilitated client for several years. Over time the client has become dependent on the case manager for emotional support and often calls the case manager. The case manager has become very fond of this client and spends more time attending to his needs than to the needs of her other clients. Finding it increasingly difficult to maintain a professional perspective, she realizes that she relates to this client as a "friend." Should this case manager continue to provide case management services to this client? Should she contact the insurance carrier, admit that her objectivity is now compromised, and have the client transferred to another nurse? Can she regain a professional level of care with this client and provide equal service to all her clients?

Clearly, the best approach is to diminish the likelihood of overinvolvement. This can be achieved by frequent, honest self-analysis. However, in the event that the nurse's objectivity becomes compromised to the point where she experiences a conflict of interest, it is wise to inform the carrier so that other personnel can be assigned.

Patient Advocate Versus Insurance Representative

Patient advocacy is central to nursing. The American Nurses Association (ANA) Code for Nurses states that the nurse is required to take action if the rights or best interests of the client are placed in jeopardy by the health care team or by the health care system.[6]

The case manager, however, wears two hats: that of patient advocate and that of insurance carrier representative. This double representation affects the external case manager more profoundly than the case manager working within a facility. Since the external case manager receives the referral from the insurance carrier, and is being paid by the carrier, it should be the primary customer. This can often result in an ethical dilemma for the case manager.

For example, a case manager is assigned to a client diagnosed with cancer which has metastasized to multiple organs. At the time of the referral the client is in an acute care facility. The insurance company's internal case manager requests on-site case management to coordinate a cost-effective discharge plan. The on-site case manager knows that the most cost-effective placement for the client would be to transfer her to a subacute facility. The client wants to go home, which would be more costly because of the amount of skilled care required. As the patient advocate, the case manager is professionally bound to abide by the client's wishes. As a representative of the insurance carrier, the case manager is expected to coordinate the most cost-effective discharge plan. What is "best" for both parties directly conflict with each other. What action to take becomes an ethical dilemma.

Confidentiality Issues

The rapport established between the client and the case manager can at times lead to overdisclosure of information (by either party), placing the case manager in a quandary about what action would be appropriate. For example, a client has sustained a back injury from a work-related accident. During the course of conversation, the client tells the case manager that she is HIV positive. She also requests that this information remain confidential. Whereas that diagnosis may affect the client's healing process, it is clearly not related to the workers' compensation claim. If the case manager includes the client's HIV status in his or her report, the client's future employment may be in jeopardy. If the HIV status goes unreported and the client has prolonged healing or costly complications following a surgical procedure, the insurance carrier would need to know this information. If the case manager informs the carrier, has he or she breached privileged information? If the case manager does not inform the carrier, is she or he performing the duties as a representative of the insurance company? The case manager has a fiduciary relationship with both the insurance carrier and the client. A *fiduciary relationship* is a legal relationship between two parties when one party relies on and trusts the other, such as between the nurse and client or the nurse and insurance company. The appropriate course of action in this particular scenario may require legal advice.

Conflict in Values

As with all nurses, case managers have their own sets of values and beliefs. At times, the case manager's philosophical belief system may directly conflict with the client's values, causing an ethical dilemma under certain circumstances. The nurse with strong religious convictions may be unable to provide unbiased care to a woman who has to contemplate aborting a pregnancy that is sure to result in a multidisabled child. The nurse providing case management to the person requesting removal of a gastrostomy tube may be faced with an ethical dilemma if the client believes that providing nutrition is beyond "extraordinary" care, and the nurse believes gastrostomy tube feeding is a basic need. An ethical dilemma may also be faced by the nurse working with a terminally ill client who continues to demand aggressive treatment despite the physician's documentation that any further treatment would be futile.

It is difficult at best to separate our personal values from our professional responsibilities. The case manager, as with all nurses, must accomplish the impossible: remain objective and nonjudgmental when working with clients whose morals and values are completely opposite to those of the nurse.

Treatment Issues with Minors

Providing services to minors can lead to triangular ethical dilemmas when the nurse believes that the parents' decisions may negatively influence the child's health status or desires. As an example, a case manager works with Mario, a 17 year old catastrophically injured in a diving accident. He sustained a C-2 spinal cord injury resulting in ventilator dependency and quadriplegia. After 6 months, the nurse and the client have developed a professional relationship based on trust. While the case manager is visiting Mario at the rehabilitation center, planning for discharge home, Mario states that he cannot live his life in his present state and requests that he be allowed to die. After many lengthy discussions with Mario, his parents, the physician, and the psychologist, it becomes evident that Mario has given this decision much thought, is mentally competent, and is prepared to end his life rather than live in his present state for possibly 50 years or more. Mario's parents completely oppose their son's wishes and state that since he is still a minor, he cannot legally decide to terminate or withdraw treatment. How should the case manager deal with this ethical dilemma? As the patient advocate, is the advocacy role compromised if she or he does not assist Mario? Or, since Mario is a minor, should the case manager align with the parents? There are no easy answers for situations such as this, and there are no right or wrong solutions.

Many times dilemmas evolve from religious beliefs versus procedures considered taboo. Ethical conflicts may arise with the Jehovah's Witness who will not allow the child to receive lifesaving transfusions; the Christian Scientist who will not administer prescribed medication; the Amish parents who have agreed to put electricity into their home so that they can keep their ventilator-dependent child at home but refuse to purchase a backup generator stating that the generator would be too extreme for compromise.

Many of these ethical dilemmas result in court decisions. However, the case manager remains central to the care and wellbeing of the child until the court decides on the appropriate action to be taken. Many internal case managers can bring their ethical dilemmas to an institutional ethics committee for discussion and resolution. The external case manager may not be as fortunate. Recently, however, more case management firms are establishing ethics committees to assist case managers.

As technology continues to expand the lifespan, as the definitions of *alive* and *living* are seen as opposite states, and as the health care system continues to ration care, ethical dilemmas will become increasingly common while remaining difficult to resolve.

LEGAL ISSUES IN CASE MANAGEMENT

Case managers are increasingly being named as defendants in lawsuits. Historically, the providers of care have carried all the risk. But, as case managers become more influential in decision making, their liability risk increases. In many instances, suits revolve around nonpayment for services that the case manager coordinated, or early discharge from an acute or subacute facility.

Standards of Care

The courts decide what is acceptable care by depending on national standards. The case manager who does not practice within accepted standards can be liable for negligence.[7] The Case Management Society of America (CMSA) has published national standards of care for the case manager. The standards specify six areas of the case manager's role: (1) assessment and case identification and selection, (2) problem identification, (3) planning, (4) monitoring, (5) evaluating, and (6) outcomes.[8]

The standards are very broad and comprehensive. They have not been tested in the courts as yet and may cause more risk than protection for the case manager. Elizabeth Hogue, BSN, JD, a health care attorney, raised several questions related to the broad scope of responsibility given by the CMSA standards:

- Are the responsibilities so broad that the case manager can be held liable for almost anything that goes wrong with the client's care?
- If an agreement regarding care cannot be reached among the patient, the family, the treatment team, and the case manager, whose recommendations will govern, specifically when the case manager is working for the payer?
- Can the standard of continuous evaluating and monitoring be interpreted to mean that the case manager is responsible for the quality of care given by all the treatment providers?
- If the patient does not reach the expected outcome, does that mean the case manager violated applicable standards of care?[9]

Who Is Liable

In order to hold case managers responsible for negligence or denial of payment, the client must prove the following:

- The case manager has a duty to make reasonable decisions or referrals.
- This duty is breached when the case manager fails to authorize payment for services deemed appropriate.
- The case manager's failure to authorize payment resulted in injury to the client.[10]

A case manager can breach her duty by "an act" or "an omission." She can either omit to do something that she should have done, or she may do something that she should not have done. To hold the case manager liable, the client must prove that the case manager committed either an act, or an omission, which resulted in injury. The courts define *causation* in terms of "but for." For example, a client states that "but for" authorization for physical therapy the injury would not have occurred.[11]

The last requirement to claim negligence is proof of injury. In most instances the courts mean physical injury. The only exception that allows emotional damages to meet the requirements of negligence is when the case manager's behavior is "extreme and outrageous." A frequently cited example of extreme and outrageous behavior does not actually involve a case manager but clearly illustrates the term. A man was in the delivery room with his wife, who died suddenly. The man put his hand on his wife's abdomen and felt fetal movement. He proceeded to plead with the providers of care in the delivery room to perform an emergency cesarean section to save the life of the infant. The physician refused. While the man continued pleading, the baby died. The providers were sued for emotional damages based on extreme and outrageous behavior. The court decided in favor of the plaintiff.[12]

Wickline v. State of California (1986) is often cited to illustrate the risk involved when making a case management decision. Briefly, this case concerns a physician who requested additional hospitalization for his patient, Lois Wickline. The hospitalization extension was denied by MediCal. Subsequently, Wickline suffered complications that necessitated amputation of her leg. She sued MediCal and was awarded $500,000. The decision was reversed in 1989, and the physician was held ultimately responsible.

The Wickline case as it pertains to case management liability has been interpreted as a caution to case managers as they are increasingly involved in patient care decisions. As case managers have greater involvement in patient decisions, their duty of care increases.[13]

Maintaining the Patient's Privacy

With the advent of the fax machine, case managers rarely mail medical documents. Unfortunately, faxing a client's medical records can place the case manager at risk for a suit for invasion of privacy. According to Kathleen Lambert, BSN, JD, a nurse attorney in Tucson, Arizona, "invasion of privacy is a violation of the right to protection against unreasonable and unwarranted interference of one's solitude, or the violation of one's right to be left alone."[14]

Although communicating with providers via phone, fax, or E-mail has become the norm, the following precautions should be taken to avoid invasion of privacy issues:

1. Never use the fax to transmit potentially harmful information, such as HIV status.
2. Always confirm the fax number and verify receipt of faxes.
3. Faxes should be reviewed and filed immediately upon receipt.[15]
4. Fax cover sheets should always include a *disclaimer,* a statement documenting that the faxed information is intended only for the person to whom it is addressed. The message should also state that the information contained in the fax is *privileged and confidential* and that any distribution or copying of the contents is strictly prohibited. Include the mailing address and/or phone number of the person transmitting the fax; that way, the person who faxed it can be notified immediately and ask the receiver to mail the communication back.

Informed Consent

The CMSA standards state that "prior to initiating the patient assessment, the case manager will define his or her role so that the patient is fully aware of and *informed* of the scope of the case manager's activities."[16] Without informed consent, a case manager increases the risk for claims of negligence.

Elizabeth Hogue, BSN, JD, raises some common concerns and criteria about the issue of informed consent:

- The two prerequisites for a valid consent are that the client is consenting voluntarily and that the client has the capacity to give consent.
- The person signing the consent must be at the age of adulthood. The age at which a person reaches adulthood is determined by state statutes. There are certain exceptions to this rule, depending on individual state laws concerning emancipation due to childbirth, or the ability to remain self-supporting.
- Informed consent involves providing the client with a specific description of the case manager's services, benefits and risks of the services, possible alternative services, and a clear statement that the services are voluntary.
- Documentation of consent is essential. This can be in the form of a signed consent form, a videotape in accordance with applicable state laws, or documentation in the patient's chart with or without the patient's signature.
- Parents, attorneys, or legal guardians may sign consent for children or incapacitated adults.[17]

Confidentiality

Disclosing confidential information can place a case manager at risk for liability. The CMSA standards state that disclosure of medical information pertaining to AIDS/HIV status, mental health records, and drug and alcohol treatment is regulated by federal and state law.[18]

Thorough documentation and a signed, informed consent serve as an excellent strategy to protect the case manager against liability for disclosure of confidential information. It is important that the nurse becomes aware of any state laws that provide specific consent form requirements for information pertaining to HIV status or to substance abuse.

In addition to receiving a signed consent, the case manager should inform the client that information may be shared with other providers. Clients should be made aware that they can refuse to sign consent forms and can withhold information; however, depending on the specific insurance coverage, refusing to disclose information may affect the case manager's ability to perform effective case management. For further protection, the case manager should document what she or he told the client and what the client responded. Every nurse should know, "If it isn't documented, it wasn't done."

Patient Assessment

Another area of concern for the case manager is the responsibility for patient assessment. To avoid a claim of negligent assessment, the case manager should review the criteria for assessment as outlined in the CMSA standards. The CMSA guidelines clearly state that the purpose of assessment is to identify the patient's individual needs. "Information is collected from a variety of sources: patient, providers, family, employer, payer."[19] The case manager should review past medical history and utilization of medical resources, understand the current diagnosis, know the expected treatment plan and expected outcomes. The case manager should identify any barriers or problems that could interfere with providing cost-effective, quality care. These may include religious or ethnic beliefs, language barriers, or absence of a support system. And of course the case manager should have a clear understanding of insurance and coverage issues as they relate to the client.[20]

How to Avoid Liability

To protect yourself from liability, develop three safety nets:

1. Design written guidelines for decision making to avoid making inconsistent decisions.
2. Establish continuous quality improvement (CQI) to ensure that the decision-making guidelines are adhered to.
3. Develop a grievance or appeals procedure for the client to use when a disagreement arises over the case manager's decision. This allows for discussion and resolution before a lawsuit is filed.[21]

In essence, to reduce the risk for liability the case manager should be familiar with the national standards and adhere to them with proper, thorough documentation, be sure that the patient has given informed consent, establish good rapport and a trusting relationship with the patient, and encourage open communication and expression, especially if there is dissatisfaction with the case management plan. The case manager must never promise what may not be possible and must ensure that the patient has a complete understanding of the services that will and will not be provided.

Chapter
Highlights

*   Case managers, as well as all health care workers, face an increasing number of ethical dilemmas as a result of advanced technology and cost-saving strategies.
*   Ethical decision making is based on 12 traditionally accepted perspectives.
*   Individuals' value systems promote adherence to different ethical perspectives. The difference in personal views may

lead to conflict between health care professionals and between health care professionals and clients.

* The case manager is faced with a multitude of ethical dilemmas. The most common ones are (1) rationing health care, (2) overinvolvement, (3) role of patient advocate versus insurance representative, (4) confidentiality issues, (5) conflict in values, and (6) treatment issues with minors.
* Case managers increasingly are finding themselves at risk for liability.
* Acceptable care is based on national standards.
* To be found liable, the claimant must prove that the case manager breached his or her duty through either "act" or "omission," the result of which was injury to the patient.
* The best protection for the case manager to reduce the risk for liability is to obtain and ensure (1) informed consent, (2) protection of privacy, (3) adherence to confidentiality statutes, (4) adherence to national standards, and (5) thorough documentation.

References

1. Clark, M. (1996). *Nursing in the community* (2d ed.). E. Norwalk, CT: Appleton & Lange. p. 259.
2. Ibid., p. 260.
3. Ibid., pp. 260–261.
4. Stanhope, M., & Lancaster, J. (1996). *Community health nursing* (4th ed.). St. Louis: Mosby. p. 95.
5. Ibid.
6. Ibid., p. 98.
7. Hogue, E. (1995, Aug.). Are case managers liable? *The Journal of Case Management.* 1(2), 36.
8. St. Coeur, M. (1996). *Case management practice guidelines.* St Louis, MO: Mosby. pp. 3–7
9. Hogue, E. (1995, June). Do CMSA standards work for or against you? *Case Management Advisor.* 6(6), 87.

10. Hogue, Are case managers liable? p. 35.

11. Ibid., p. 36.

12. Hogue, E. (1995, Mar.). CMs beware! Legal spotlight turns to CM. *Case Management Advisor*. 6(3), 43.

13. Hyatt, T. (1994, July–Aug.–Sept.). Legal hazards on the case management highway. *The Case Manager*. 5(3), 102, 111.

14. Lambert, K. (1995, Nov.). 13 tips help cms keep patient records safe. *Case Management Advisor*. 6(11), 158.

15. Ibid., p. 159.

16. St. Coeur, *Case management practice guidelines*. p. 3.

17. Hogue, Elizabeth. (1995, May). Tips make CMSA standards work for you. *Case Management Advisor*. 6(5), 75–76.

18. St. Coeur, *Case management practice guidelines*. p. 12

19. Ibid., p. 4.

20. Ibid.

21. Hogue, Are case managers liable? pp. 38–39.

Populations with 11
Special Needs

A client diagnosed with HIV/AIDS or mental illness has needs that may not be entirely met using traditional models of case management. The chronicity of these diseases, social stigma, issues of confidentiality, and lack of agreement in the medical community or absence of effective treatment are only a few of the issues that influence the case management process.

High-risk maternity, neonatal, and pediatric case management also create special issues. With advances in technology, low-birth-weight babies, as well as newborns with multiple anomalies and/or complications, are surviving. Even 10 or 15 years ago these infants would have died shortly after birth. Now, they may spend months in neonatal intensive care units and often require a lifetime of complex medical care attention. Technology has allowed severely brain injured or spinal-cord-injured children and teenagers to live, recover, and in many instances reenter the community as productive citizens. The case management process specific to these populations must be multidisciplinary, collaborative, and comprehensive, since management may extend for several years or more. The case manager must also remain aware that there are two clients: the injured child and the family.

This chapter explores many of the problems encountered and some solutions for those problems when providing case management services to these clients. Upon completion of this chapter you will be able to answer the following questions:

1. How do the needs of clients with HIV/AIDS influence the role of the case manager?
2. How do the needs of clients with mental illness influence the role of the case manager?
3. How can effective case management alter outcomes for high-risk pregnant women?
4. What are the problems unique to low-birth-weight and/or medically compromised newborns and children with long-term care needs?

CLIENTS WITH HIV/AIDS

When case management was in its infancy, client selection for case management targeted cases in which high-dollar claims were anticipated. Through early identification, appropriate and cost-effective care could be coordinated in a timely fashion. Case management was episodic and focused on resolving the current crisis.

The criteria for early identification were usually established through *ICD-9 codes* (the statistical classification that organizes diseases and injuries into groups according to standardized criteria). Case management strategies focused on facilitating the client's transfer to a step-down unit or to a less costly alternative setting. When the crisis was resolved, the case manager terminated the relationship and closed the case. If another crisis erupted, the case manager was called in again, and the cycle was repeated.

With the onset of the AIDS epidemic, it soon became evident that clients who might benefit from case management could no longer be identified through ICD-9 coding alone. Physicians, concerned about issues of confidentiality, used the diagnosis that was the immediate reason for hospital admission, such as pneumonia or diarrhea, rather than the ICD-9 code for AIDS. True stories of employees terminated from their workplace when their diagnosis of AIDS became known added to physicians' hesitancy to document diagnosis.

Since the early 1990s legislation regarding confidentiality issues has eased the problem of case identification. It soon became evident that the cost of treating AIDS was devastating not only to the health care system but to the individual as well. "The first 10,000 cases accounted for 1.6 million days of in patient hospitalization at a cost of $1.4 billion."[1] The recent discovery that protease inhibitors, in combination with existing anti-HIV therapy, can halt the spread of the virus into healthy cells has led researchers to believe that the treatment of AIDS has entered a new phase. However, this treatment can cost between $12,000 and $18,000 per year. Add to that the multiple medications used to treat related complications and the bill can rise to $70,000 per year.[2] *This amount is for medication only.* Costs for hospitalization, skilled nursing care, and/or hospice raise the bill to astronomical levels. The annual cost of treating AIDS can be $100,000 or more. The client with an 80/20 insurance policy is responsible for 20 percent of the cost. That translates into $20,000 per year out-of-pocket. Most people are unable to afford their 20 percent and seek alternative sources of financial assistance, placing a tremendous burden on federal, state, and local resources.

As case management has shifted from episodic control of a crisis to a continuous process focusing on prevention and empowerment, and as HIV/AIDS has evolved into a chronic, manageable disease state, the need for case management, cost containment, and prevention of major opportunistic infections has grown exponentially.

Understanding HIV/AIDS

Human immunodeficiency virus (HIV) is defined as an "infection caused by several related retroviruses that become incorporated into host cell DNA and result in a wide range of clinical presentations varying from asymptomatic carrier states to debilitating and fatal disorders."[3] The Centers for Disease Control and Prevention (CDC) use a classification system of nine categories to define acquired immunodeficiency syndrome (AIDS). The classification definition is as follows:

Laboratory evidence of HIV infection *plus* laboratory evidence of severe immunosuppression:

- Less than 200 CD4 + T-lymphocytes or
- CD4 + T-lymphocytes less than 14 percent of total lymphocytes

and/or one or more of 26 clinical conditions meeting AIDS surveillance case definition (see Table 11-1).

AIDS related complex (ARC) is a term previously used to describe a constellation of signs and symptoms found in some persons infected with HIV. "Most of the clinical findings which were formally denoted as ARC are now in groups 3 or 4 of the CDC AIDS classification system."[4]

HIV retroviruses decimate part of the body's immune system by destroying CD4 + lymphocytes, considered the first line of defense against any virus entering the body.

Table 11-1. Clinical Conditions Necessary for AIDS Surveillance[5]

Candidiasis of bronchi, trachea, or lungs	Kaposi's sarcoma
Candidiasis, esophageal	Lymphoma (Burkitt's; immuno-blastic; primary in brain)
Coccidiomycosis, disseminated or extrapulmonary	Mycobacterium
Cryptococcosis, extrapulmonary	Pneumocystis carinii pneumonia
Cryptosporidiosis, chronic intestinal (> 1-month duration)	Progressive multifocal leuko-encephalopathy
Cytomegalovirus disease (other than liver, spleen or nodes)	Salmonella septicemia, recurrent
Cytomegalovirus retinitis (with loss of vision)	Toxoplasmosis of brain
HIV encephalopathy	Wasting syndrome due to HIV
Herpes simplex: Chronic ulcer(s)	Pulmonary tuberculosis
	Recurrent pneumonia (bacterial, more than 1 episode)
	Invasive cervical cancer

Normally there are 1000 to 1300 CD4+ cells per cubic milli-meter of blood. When the CD4+ number falls to below 200 per cubic millimeter of blood, the immune system begins to fail, and the person is diagnosed with AIDS.[6]

Current available drugs such as AZT work by suppressing the replication of HIV.[7] However, mutations often occur when HIV replicates, rendering HIV resistant to AZT and other anti-HIV drugs. Protease, an enzyme in the HIV virus, is essential for viral replication. Recent research with protease inhibitors is promising, since the drug inhibits the HIV enzyme and prevents the formation of new HIV mutations.[8]

Issues and Treatment Options

Since AIDS was first recognized in 1981, approximately 500,000 cases in the United States have been reported. It is estimated that an additional unreported 1 million people are infected with HIV.[9] In the early years a diagnosis of AIDS was a death sentence. Most people diagnosed as HIV+ had full blown AIDS within 2 years. Treatment was aimed at limiting the occurrence of opportunistic infections and lengthy hospitalization stays.

Ignorance and prejudice resulted in overwhelming fear among the private as well as the professional sectors. Persons with AIDS (PWAs) were abandoned by their support systems and became financially and emotionally drained.

Through medical research and intensive educational programs, people are beginning to realize that although AIDS has reached epi-demic proportions, it is preventable and treatable as well as con-trollable for longer periods. The changing demographics of the epidemic have decreased the judgmental and homophobic reactions of many health care providers. It is well known that AIDS cuts across both genders, all ages, all economic levels, and all ethnicities. Unfortunately, too many professionals still cling to the obsolete concept of high-risk groups and a belief system that blames the vic-tim. I have known nurse case managers as well as physicians who refused to drink out of a well-washed glass in the home of a client with AIDS despite their knowledge that the disease is not transmitted through casual contact.

More than for any other disease entity, nurse case managers working with clients diagnosed with HIV or AIDS must examine their own feelings toward sexuality, homosexuality, and death. Because of the multiple clinical problems that the HIV infected person may present with, nurse case managers must thoroughly understand the process of the disease and common symptomatology. They must keep up with recent drug therapies, attend conferences, and review the literature on a regular basis. Because of the devastating financial drain on clients diagnosed with AIDS, the case manager must maintain a thorough resource file containing support groups; federal, state, and local services; and current trends in research and legislation. (See Appendix II for a list of resources related to HIV/AIDS.)

Remember too that many clients diagnosed with HIV/AIDS are often extremely knowledgeable about the disease process and recent drug therapies. With most other diagnoses, a large part of the case management process is educating the client. With AIDS, the client may have the most recent information about research and pharmaceutical trials.

The Ungvarski Management Program

As more clients with HIV/AIDS are treated as outpatients, the need for effective case management has increased. Many case management firms have developed models for the client with HIV/AIDS. One such model has been designed by Peter J. Ungvarski, MS, RN, FAAN, clinical director of AIDS services for the Visiting Nurse Service of New York.

When working with patients diagnosed with AIDS, a comprehensive case management approach must encompass more than coordination of cost-effective care. Programs must be included that try to reduce the spread of HIV. Prevention saves lives and reduces the rising costs of treating the diagnosis.

Ungvarski has designed a three-tiered case management program for clients with HIV/AIDS. He outlines the main concerns of health care delivery as primary, secondary, and tertiary prevention.

In the Ungvarski model, the focus of primary prevention is identification of people whose behavior places them at risk, determination of the need for education to reduce risk behavior, and detection of signs and symptoms suggestive of HIV infection or AIDS. Primary prevention includes taking a thorough health history with emphasis on risk behavior. A comprehensive social and sexual history is essential to detect potential or actual HIV exposure.

Too often, many health care providers erroneously believe that people over 50 do not engage in high-risk sexual behaviors. However, HIV and other sexually transmitted diseases are increasing in the elderly population. "The inability of primary care providers to suspect HIV infection in older clients has led to misdiagnosis of Alzheimer's disease in the presence of HIV encephalopathy and has delayed the diagnosis of pneumonia caused by *Pneumocystis carinii* (PCP) in elderly individuals."[10]

Secondary prevention is aimed at empowering HIV-infected clients to manage their own care. An enlightened case manager will realize that effective planning should be deferred until the client has adjusted to a recent diagnosis. Despite increased lifespan through appropriate treatment and possibly decades between the initial diagnosis of HIV and a diagnosis of AIDS, most newly diagnosed clients may feel hopeless, depressed, panicked, and suicidal.

Once the client has come to terms with the diagnosis, the case manager can begin designing a plan of care with the client. The initial plan should include education about health-promoting activities. Current research in the area of behaviors that have positive effects on the immune system are promising.[11] Strong evidence suggests enhanced immune system function in people who are exposed to humor, creative imagery, and positive thinking. However, too many health care delivery professionals are unfamiliar with how to help the client effect changes in behavior. If a physician or a nurse tells a client what to do, they assume that the "compliant" client will automatically do as told.

Other areas of secondary prevention include:

1. Follow-up physician appointments to assess immune system status
2. Prophylactic drug therapy
3. Immunizations and vaccinations
4. Evaluating HIV-infected women for pregnancy, with appropriate medication to reduce the risk of mother to child transmission.

Tertiary prevention focuses on minimizing the occurrence of opportunistic infections. Medication treatments available today can suppress or control the occurrence of many common infections. Such treatments can increase the client's quality of life, maximize independence, and save thousands of health care dollars. For example, Atavoquone can be used to treat PCP and practically eliminates the need for hospitalization.[12]

Ungvarski indicates three major problem areas that the case manager confronts in the process of developing an effective care plan:

- The amount of medications that the client will need to take on a daily basis is increasing. A large percentage of clients need assistance, supervision, or reminders to ensure proper administration.
- Underdiagnosed cognitive impairment can result in an inability of the client to carry out the plan of care. Studies indicate that although many physicians do not diagnose cognitive problems until the advanced stages, nurses and other caregivers have reported memory deficits much earlier in the disease process.
- The primary physician may not document continued drug abuse and alcoholism. Mixing alcohol with some of the anti-HIV medications can result in serious or life-threatening side effects.[13]

In essence, this model of case management incorporates education, behavior modification, control of symptoms, and empowering clients to manage their own care. When successful, such a program can increase the client's quality of life and independence and decrease costly complications while saving millions of health care dollars.

Financial Support

Medicaid is the main source of public funding for people with AIDS. It is estimated that 40 to 70 percent of HIV-infected people receive assistance through Medicaid programs.[14] Other sources of assistance include:

- *Social Security Disability Insurance (SSDI).* This federal program, operated through the Social Security Administration, provides monthly benefits to physically or mentally disabled workers who have paid into social security. The amount of benefits paid is based on the person's earnings history. The disabled worker must prove that the disability will last for at least one year, or that the impairment is expected to be fatal.
- *Social Security Income (SSI).* This federal welfare program is operated through the Social Security Administration and provides income to low-income, aged, blind, and disabled people.
- *Aid to Families with Dependent Children (AFDC).* This federal-state welfare program provides monthly benefits to people with at least one child under the age of 18. Each state establishes eligibility criteria. For the most part income thresholds below 50 percent of the poverty level are required. Many states deny coverage if two parents reside in the home, and almost 90 percent of AFDC recipients are single female parents.[15]
- *General Assistance (GA).* Most, but not all, states operate a GA program that provide benefits to those who do not qualify for AFDC and who are not yet disabled long enough to collect from SSI.
- *Department of Veterans Affairs (VA).* This federally funded program provides benefits to veterans who have served in the armed forces for at least 180 days and who have received an honorable or general discharge. Although first priority is

given to veterans whose disability is service related, funds may be available for non-service-related disabilities.

Additional resources to explore include: community outreach programs, private charities, employer long-term disability programs, the recently developed viatical settlements, and accelerated death benefits (ADB). A *viatical settlement* allows people facing life-threatening illnesses to sell their life insurance policies to a third party for cash. The company purchasing the policy becomes the beneficiary and pays all future premiums to keep the policy in force. ADB is more restrictive than viatical settlements but remains an option for the financially drained client.

It is likely that the case manager working with people diagnosed with HIV/AIDS will need to assist the client in tapping resources for financial assistance. Eligibility requirements differ from resource to resource and, at times, from state to state. The case manager must maintain current information regarding the various services, eligibility requirements, and appropriate referral sources.

Confidentiality Issues

Due to fear of termination by their employers or ostracism from the community, many people infected with HIV are hesitant to discuss their diagnosis. As a result, establishing rapport with clients diagnosed with HIV may be more difficult than usual. The case manager must be sensitive to the client's fears and must also be aware of government guidelines concerning disclosure of information.

Confidentiality issues play an important role when caregivers are involved. Some state laws prohibit disclosure of HIV status without permission from the client. This means that explaining universal precautions and procedures to a caregiver could be viewed as a masked approach to discussing the client's diagnosis. Since the case manager may not be permitted to discuss the client's HIV status, she or he will need to be creative in finding ways to educate the caregiver regarding health safety and still maintain the client's confidentiality.

Currently, statutes of each state specify the parameters of what information can be disclosed and to whom it can be given. However, the Medical Records Confidentiality Act, if passed by Congress, will establish uniform federal guidelines for the use and disclosure of medical information. One major problem with this proposed enactment of federal legislation will be the establishment of large computer databases, which corporate America will be able to purchase. The current bill does not require that the patient be informed when the records become part of a database.

Increased access to medical records through large computer databases can have serious consequences to people infected with HIV/AIDS, as well as those diagnosed with mental illness.

MENTAL ILLNESS

Before the 1960s, people with mental illness were afforded few rights. With the enactment of mental health codes, people with mental illness were guaranteed the same basic rights as the general population. Despite legislation, a diagnosis of mental illness still carries with it social stigma in the general community and often a lack of understanding within the professional community. Unlike a fractured arm, mental illness cannot be seen, cannot be examined under a microscope, and often cannot be described in scientifically objective terminology.

Mental illness is neither obscure nor rare. It is estimated that "in any given year, more than five million Americans suffer from an acute episode of mental illness such as schizophrenia, manic depression, severe depression, obsessive-compulsive disorder, and panic disorder. One in five families in the United States is directly affected by one of these disorders in their lifetime."[16] When addictive disorder is added, the number of affected people jumps to over 80 million.[17]

Mental illness is costly, debilitating, and misunderstood. In the past, those diagnosed with mental illness were institutionalized, often for decades. However, within the past 10 to 15 years, medical and pharmaceutical research, in combination with high-tech diagnostic equipment, have resulted in significantly improved treatment for the mentally ill. People with a diagnosis such as bipolar disorder (i.e., manic depression) or schizophrenia, previously considered untreatable, can often be treated with drug therapy. The person suffering with schizophrenia or bipolar disorder who takes the prescribed medication can function within society with little problem. These medications have not only increased the client's ability to function but also have virtually eliminated much of the high cost of other forms of treatment. For example, during one 10-year period the use of lithium as a treatment for manic depression saved an estimated $2.8 billion in medical costs.[18]

Issues

A huge problem when working with clients diagnosed with mental illness is a lack of adequate insurance coverage. Most insurance companies, whether traditional indemnity or managed care, put a limit on outpatient treatment and often have stringent coverage restrictions. Coverage is mandated by states and varies from state to state. These limits often result in financial devastation to the client and family—as well as an additional burden on community and government resources.

The National Alliance for the Mentally Ill (NAMI)—currently numbering approximately 140,000 members—has recently started a campaign calling for changes in public and private policies that have negative impact on people with mental illness. NAMI has highlighted a study that indicates identical prevalence of epilepsy and schizophrenia; however, health insurers provide full coverage to people diagnosed with epilepsy and leave "tens of thousands of people with schizophrenia reliant on public assistance for access to life saving treatment."[19] The report states that "both diagnoses are brain disorders, affect one in 100 people, are chronic conditions that may be life threatening, and yet can be successfully treated."[20]

Mental Illness and Case Management

Mental illness encompasses much more than the diagnoses of psychoses listed above. Physical and mental health are often interrelated. Depression, anxiety, and/or panic may accompany a diagnosis of cancer, AIDS, or other catastrophic illness. Too often the primary physician overlooks the mental disorder and treats only the physical problem. Unfortunately, this means only half the client is treated. Positive outcomes will be less than expected without an holistic approach.

Posttraumatic stress disorder (PTSD) is a common diagnosis following a traumatic event. If left untreated, the person will likely return to the emergency room or to the primary physician with repeated somatic complaints. Costly diagnostic tests will be performed to rule out organic causes. If the root of the problem is never touched on, the client remains symptomatic, unable to function independently within society, unproductive at best at work, and the subject of continued, rising medical costs.

Panic disorder is another condition that may be undiagnosed as it mimics many cardiac conditions. The patient will complain of shortness of breath, chest pain, palpitations, and anxiety. Without proper and comprehensive assessment, the misdiagnosed client undergoes unnecessary and expensive cardiac testing.

According to Thomas N. Wise, MD, professor and vice chairman of the Department of Psychiatry at Georgetown University in Washington, DC, "25 percent to 30 percent of all patients admitted to primary care facilities have hidden mental disorders."[21] With appropriate and timely psychiatric assessment, early diagnosis and treatment will reduce the cost of medical care.

Case managers must play a pivotal role in assessing and coordinating follow-up treatment when the possibility of underlying mental disorders exists. Often, it is the case manager who first recognizes that physical symptoms might be secondary to psychological problems and who therefore can facilitate communication among the primary physician, the psychiatrist, and/or the social worker as well as family members or other support systems. The case manager can provide emotional support, refer the client to appropriate resources, and help the family understand and participate willingly for the best outcome for the client.

It is within the case manager's sphere of duties to convince the insurance carrier to provide the appropriate treatment. This may include going out of contract and covering extended psychiatric or substance abuse therapy, since large dollar savings can be achieved by avoiding the physical or medical complications that may crop up without proper treatment and follow-up. A person with recurrent suicidal ideation, for example, may attempt suicide in any number of ways, including self-mutilation; motor vehicle accidents; or overdosing on drugs, alcohol, or some combination that can lead to severe brain damage which can cost a lifetime of treatment and care.

Another problem with clients with mental illness is that they are often noncompliant with medication treatment, which can lead to high readmission rates. Some home care agencies have developed *psychiatric home health services* to address this issue. The case manager, collaborating with the home care agency, can show the carrier that providing home care services increases compliance and decreases hospital recidivism. Since the cost for inpatient psychiatric care averages $600 to $800 per day on a national basis and the average cost for a home visit by a psychiatric nurse averages between $65 and $95 per visit, the numbers should be convincing.[22]

A problem unique to case managers working with clients injured in work-related accidents involves appropriate treatment of stress syndromes. Workers' compensation insurance benefits covers all expenses directly related to an injury. A work-injured client who is also diagnosed with PTSD will receive appropriate psychiatric treatment for the duration of that physical injury. Problems arise when the psychiatrist recommends continued treatment for psychiatric problems that may or may not be related to the injury. A physician can easily determine that a knee injury sustained weeks later is unrelated to the work injury. However, it is often impossible for the psychiatrist to categorize client's emotional problems. For example, a client involved in a chemical explosion at work

challenges to the nurse case manager. When providing help to medically unstable infants, the case manager has two clients—the infant and the family members. The goal for such infants is to stabilize the medical status and to empower the family to partake in the child's care. The long-term objective is to enable families to become their own case managers.

Before the high-tech equipment available today was developed, most very low-birth-weight neonates did not survive. Now, a large percentage of these children become medically stable and are discharged from the acute care setting. Unfortunately, many survivors have delayed developmental progress, learning disabilities, medical complications, and lifelong disabilities. With appropriate management and rehabilitation, a significant number of these children can be mainstreamed into school and into the community as they grow.

The case management process begins with facilitating communication between the parents, the physician, the NICU nurses, and the insurance carrier. Positive outcomes for children who will have lifelong medical problems and complications depends on the family's ability to adjust to, accept, and bond with the newborn as early as possible. The family problems—including financial stress, marital discord, and decreased time available for the other children in the family—can have serious consequences. Professionals now realize that providing psychosocial assistance to the family as a whole is as important as providing medical care to the child. This is especially true when the primary caregiver is employed full-time.

When the infant is medically stable enough for discharge from the acute care facility, the case manager is central in developing a plan of care with the family and providers of care. Coordinating appropriate, cost-effective home care and providing information about community resources and government assistance programs enable many parents to care for their child at home rather than in a long-term care facility.

A viable discharge plan includes coordination with: (1) alternative caregivers, (2) a local pharmacy, (3) appropriate physicians, perhaps a neonatologist, a pediatric pulmonologist, or a pediatric physiatrist, (4) home care agencies specializing in neonatal and pediatric care, (5) provider of DME and supplies, and (6) when appropriate, referral to the local Women, Infant and Children (WIC) site, for nutritional assistance.

Many parents are emotionally, physically, or financially unable to care for their medically dependent child at home. Throughout the country, long-term care facilities provide cost-effective, quality care. It is the responsibility of the case manager to educate the parents about the different options available and to provide enough information to clarify any misconceptions regarding long-term care facilities. The programs available today for children are vastly different from the dreary institutions of years ago. Facilities today offer a nurturing environment, aggressive and maintenance therapy, education by teachers who are certified in special education, and group trips to various local recreational sites.

For the child who is cared for at home, the case manager can coordinate enrollment into a medical day care program. Most states offer programs with a stimulating environment for the child. These programs give respite to the primary caregiver, allow the parent to return to work, and afford medical surveillance and socialization for the child.

Case managing infants and children must be continuously revised as the child grows. The ultimate goal is to provide enough education, information, emotional and psychosocial assistance, and referral sources so that the family can take on the job of case managing the child. Throughout the process, the case manager must try to avoid a common pitfall—becoming too emotionally attached to the child and the family—as this can foster dependency on the part of the family members.

PEDIATRIC AND TEENAGE REHAB

As with the low-birth-weight infant, technology today has extended the lifespan of the severely head- or spinal-cord-injured child and adolescent. As a result of diving accidents and motor vehicle accidents, many young survivors can anticipate a lifetime of ventilator dependence. Ten to fifteen years ago, the majority of children who sustained an injury of this severity did not survive.

An overwhelming challenge for the case manager is to assist the patient and the family to accept and adjust to the drastic changes in lifestyle. The parents must revise their expectations for their child and their own goals for the future. When the injury occurs during adolescence, the usual problems associated with normal puberty are compounded.

During the time immediately following the injury, the client's friends usually rally. As time passes and the client is unable to join in the recreational and social activities of peers, the client's circle of friends gradually diminishes. The case management process can help the client to find new ways of socializing and of meeting people who have experienced similar physical and/or cognitive limitations.

Psychological counseling must be an essential and integral part of the care plan so clients can successfully integrate themselves back into the community. The case manager can coordinate psychosocial assistance to enhance the client's and the family's ability to cope with the loss of previous goals and expectations. If the insurance carrier is unwilling to extend benefit packages to include intensive, long-term counseling, coordination with community resources is essential. Psychological assistance is often needed during specific stages of development, especially during puberty when the injured client is affected by issues of sexuality and by the developmental need for peer group approval.

Since case management for the pediatric and adolescent population may continue for many years, many issues not seen with the adult client must be addressed. The plan of care will need revision as the child advances through the developmental stages. If the child is able to be mainstreamed in school, assessing the availability of a school nurse or coordinating an attendant to assist the child may be necessary. Many school districts are afraid of liability issues, which must be seen to before the child's entry into school.[26]

When working with clients with special needs, the case management process can be both challenging and rewarding. Case managers face multiple obstacles, which demand creativity, extensive knowledge, sensitivity, and empathy, as well as the best use of limited resources. They may work with a client and family for many years, from beginning acceptance, to mainstreaming in school, and finally to integrating into the community, at a maximum level of independence and functioning.

Chapter Highlights

* Case management models may differ depending on whether one is working with clients diagnosed with HIV/AIDS, mental illness, high-risk pregnancies, low-birth-weight babies, and/or severely injured children.
* Clients with HIV/AIDS or mental illness are often financially devastated due to the high cost of treatment and/or insurance limitations.
* Confidentiality issues can pose a complex challenge for the case manager when working with clients diagnosed with HIV/AIDS or mental illness.
* The Ungvarski model of case management developed for the client with HIV/AIDS involves comprehensive programs for three levels of prevention—identification, empowerment, and minimization.
* A large portion of the psychiatric case manager's role is to assess underlying mental illness with the client who presents with physical complaints. Through facilitating communication among the providers, she or he coordinates appropriate care using an holistic approach.
* The obstetric case manager's role is primarily educating the client and providing appropriate care through creative case management. The goal of obstetric case management is the delivery of a full-term healthy baby.
* The pediatric case manager works with the parents as well as the child. His or her role involves providing support and creating an environment conducive to bonding, family participation, and eventual integration into the community.

*   The ultimate goal for case managers working with clients who have special needs is to provide enough support, information, and education so that clients can assume the role of case manager for their own care.

References

1. Thorn, K. (1990). *Applying medical case management: AIDS.* Canoga Pk, CA: Thorn. p. 2.
2. Altman, L. (1996, Feb.). New AIDS therapies arise, but who can afford the bill? *The New York Times.* p. 1
3. Berkow, R., & Fletcher, A. (1992). *The Merck manual of diagnosis and therapy* (16th ed.). Merck Research Laboratories, Rahway, NJ. p. 77.
4. Hogan, C., & University of Minnesota. (1995, Oct.15). AIDS glossary of medical and statistical terms. *Glossary of medical, statistical, and clinical research terminology.* p. 5. [on-line]
5. Basics of HIV/AIDS Knowledge or "AIDS 101." (1996, Feb.19). *How a case of AIDS is determined.* p. 2. [on-line]
6. Berkow & Fletcher, *Merck manual.* p. 78.
7. Hogan & University of Minnesota, AIDS glossary. p. 6.
8. Ibid., pp. 45, 46.
9. Ungvarski, Peter. (1995, Oct.) Adults and HIV/AIDS: Clinical considerations for care management. *The Journal of Care Management.* 1(3), 40.
10. Ibid., p. 45.
11. Ibid., p. 49.
12. Ibid., p. 58.
13. Ibid., pp. 58–59.
14. Thorn, *Applying medical case management: AIDS.* p. 83.
15. Smith, C., & Maurer, F. (1995). *Community health nursing: Theory and practice.* Philadelphia, PA: WB Saunders. p. 125.
16. On-line psychological services (1996, Feb. 19).
17. Hoffman, L. (ed.). (1995, Jan.). Case managers who quickly spot mental disorders can reduce medical costs. *Case Management Advisor.* 6(1), 1.
18. On-line psychological services (1996, Feb.5).
19. On-line psychological services (1996, Feb.19).

20.   On-line psychological services (1996, Feb.19).

21.   Hoffman, Case managers who quickly spot mental disorders. p. 1.

22.   Hoffman, L. (ed). (1995, July). Relapse rates drop when mental health goes home. *Case Management Advisor*. 6(7), 101.

23.   Ibid., p. 89.

24.   Ibid., p. 90.

25.   Foust, R., & Norvell, J. (1996, Winter). Maternity risk management. *Case Review*. 2(1), 37.

26.   Gerson, V. (1996, Winter). Pediatric case management. *Case Review*. 2(1), 20.

Reports I

This appendix includes samples of reports that an external case manager would forward to an insurance carrier on a monthly basis. Included are examples of initial, progress, and closure reports for the client with traditional indemnity insurance and the client injured in a work-related accident.

As you read these reports, the main differences you will notice are that the health insurance company wants information regarding the client's medical status, creative planning efforts to avoid complications, and cost savings generated through case management services. The workers' compensation insurance company needs information regarding the client's vocational abilities and potential to return to work.

Although there is no universal format for reports, these examples include the necessary information required. For further amplification, refer back to Chapter 4.

The following is an appendix outline:

A. Client with traditional indemnity insurance
    1. Initial report
    2. Progress report
    3. Closure report

B. Client with workers' compensation insurance
    1. Initial report
    2. Progress report
    3. Closure report

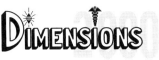

in Managed Care

INSURANCE COMPANY   **September 29, 19XX**

CLIENT	: Sylvia Thompson	**DOL: 19XX**
POLICY #	: 1234567	**DOB: 3/1/XX**
DIMENSIONS # :	148	**SS# : 222-22-2222**

DIAGNOSIS: Multiple Sclerosis

INITIAL REPORT

History of Loss

This client was referred for an initial evaluation and medical case management. With account[1] approval, this consultant conducted an initial assessment at the client's home on 10/3/XX.

In addition to the client, the client's husband and home health aide were present throughout the interview. The client remained cooperative and friendly, and answered all questions openly and honestly.

This 43-year-old female was diagnosed with multiple sclerosis in 19X0 at the age of 30. She remained stable with minimal symptomatology until 19X4. At that time she began to experience lower extremity weakness

---

[1]"Account" refers to the insurance company

and began using an AMIGO.[2] The client continued working full time until September 19X7.

Since 19X7, the client has progressed slowly through the disease process. During the early part of 19X9, the client spent 4 weeks as an inpatient at Western Rehabilitation Center. Upon discharge to home, the client privately hired a home health aide to assist with activities of daily living (ADLs). The aide provided services for 4 hours in the morning and 1 hour in the evening. This arrangement currently continues.

Until April 19X1, the client remained at home without medical complications. Since that time, she has developed pneumonia four times. On four of these occasions, hospitalization has been necessary. Since January 19X2, the client has become dependent on the use of a nebulizer machine, used three to four times daily.

The client stated that she has had decubiti in the past, which have been easily treated at home. In June 19X2, the client stated that she began to have skin breakdown at the sacral area. She was treated at home, as usual, and stated that healing appeared to be taking place slowly. In August, when there were still signs of breakdown, the client sought medical assistance with Dr. Baker, a neurologist. Dr. Baker recommended bed rest for 1 month. During that time the client developed pneumonia again, which resulted in hospitalization.

When the client was discharged, the decubitus had not yet completely healed. Treatment consisted of application of duoderm. Throughout that period, the client remained in her wheelchair for most of the day. In January 19X3, the client purchased a tilt wheelchair, which relieves pressure to sensitive areas. Due to the extent of damage already existing at the sacral area, the decubitus continued to cause problems.

In June 19X3, the client developed an infection at the decubitus site and was hospitalized for 2 weeks. Treatment consisted of debridement and IV antibiotics. Upon discharge, it was recommended that the client use an antipressure mattress, which was authorized by the insurance company and purchased through a local supplier. At about this time an occupational therapist specializing in seating became involved in the client's care. She has been assisting her with a sitting schedule and in designing a chair that will give the client the highest decubitus prevention level.

---

[2]AMIGO is a motorized scooter for mobility

Current Medical Status

At this time the client is completely dependent for all activities of daily living. She is only able to move her right hand and arm. She is unable to turn independently in bed. The client is also beginning to experience head and neck weakness and is unable to maintain her head in proper alignment. It is evident that within the very near future, a head rest will be necessary for the tilt wheelchair.

Currently the decubitus has healed. The site is clean, dry, and intact, with minimal redness. The skin is extremely fragile and needs assessment at a minimum of every 2 to 3 hours. The sitting schedule, as devised by the occupational therapist, increases by 15-minute increments daily. At this time, the client is sitting in the chair for 5 hours per day. The therapist is not going to increase above 5 hours until the skin has toughened.

The client's home care at this time includes a home health aide for 2 hours in the morning and 2 hours in the evening, which the client pays for out-of-pocket. Central Nursing Agency is providing a home health aide for an additional 4 hours daily, which is being paid for by the insurance company. The aide assesses the client's skin status prior to getting her out of bed. She then transfers the client to the tilt chair for the prescribed amount of time. She assists the client with the nebulizer treatment, meal preparation, and other ADLs. Prior to leaving, the aide transfers the client back to bed, assesses the skin status, and positions the client on her side. The aide also performs passive range of motion exercises. It was recommended and approved that the home health aide continue providing services for another 4 to 6 weeks to prevent further skin breakdown and/or complications. This case manager negotiated the cost of the home health aide to $13.50 per hour. The regular rate was quoted at $15.00 per hour.

The occupational therapist has visited the client on only six or seven occasions. The majority of her assistance is via the phone. She charges $100 per session (phone contact is not charged). Each visit requires several hours.

The client uses a foley catheter with a leg bag. She is maintained on a bowel program and retains bowel control. This consultant is in the process of assessing current cost of the catheters and other disposables. During the next report period, cost-effective coordination of disposables is a goal. Other equipment in use includes a hoyer lift, which has been purchased.

The client began to complain of exacerbation of symptoms several weeks ago. The physician recommended a 5-day Solumedrol IV treatment plan, to begin October 1, 19X3 through October 5, 19X3. This consultant coordinated the IV infusion through DEF Home Care. The IV treatment, along with nursing care, was quoted at $325.00 per day. Total cost of the treatment would be $1625.00. This consultant was given a negotiated rate of $200.00 per day, all-inclusive. The actual cost of the infusion was $1000.00. This resulted in a savings of $625.00.

Current Medications

Cardizem: 180mg. daily
Prednisone: 30mg. daily
Vitamin C: 500mg. daily

The client is very thin, with obvious atrophy of all major muscles. All physical therapy, which includes range of motion, is performed by the home health aide.

Medical History

The client states a history of hypertension since age 23. She has been treated medically and remains stable.

Socioeconomic

The client lives in a small, two-bedroom apartment in a moderately high crime area in New York. Her apartment is on the first floor of a building without an elevator; however, the entry into the building is wheelchair accessible. The client lives with her husband, who has remained out of work since he sustained a severe back injury in a work-related accident 3 years ago. Prior to his injury he had been employed as a laborer for a large construction company.

Due to the husband's medical problems, he is unable to assist with many of the client's needs. The client has no children.

The client and her husband have little knowledge and understanding regarding the disease process. This consultant suggested joining a local MS support group; however, both the client and her husband stated they had been to one support group meeting several years ago and felt that it was "not for them."

Until this recent problem with the decubitus, they have maintained independence in the coordination of the client's care. It appears that they are very motivated to return to that level. The client stated that prior to this recent complication, she was able to be alone for many hours of the day. She is anxious to return to a level where, once positioned properly in the tilt chair, she can remain seated for much of the day and return to her normal daily routine.

The client stated that she is finding it increasingly difficult to manage financially. Her husband's workers' compensation settlement, along with her long-term disability income, does not leave much additional money for non-essential expenses.

Vocational Status

The client had worked as a receptionist/secretary for a large corporation for many years. She had to retire on long-term disability in 19X7, due to her diagnosis.

Physician

Dr. Alexander Baker, Neurologist—MS specialist
000 First Street
Brooklyn, NY

(718) 111-1111

Therapist

Ellen Rodriguez, seating specialist
(718) 222-2222

Impressions / Summary

The client is a triplegic with total dependency on ADLs. She appears extremely motivated to maintain as much independence as possible. She had been independent in her daily routine until the recent development of a sacral decubitus. At this time the decubitus is healed, but the skin is very fragile.

It is this consultant's opinion that if the home care is left in place for several more weeks, prevention of major complications will be seen. If the client's skin breaks down again, the next step would be pressure mapping, which is an expensive procedure. In addition, the possibility of a skin graft remains, which would cost approximately $10,000, all-inclusive.

Due to the disease process, the client's status will continue to deteriorate. It is this consultant's opinion that large savings and quality care can be seen by providing the appropriate preventive care at this time.

It is also this consultant's opinion that the client and her husband need education regarding the disease and the disease process. This is important for them to be able to make informed decisions regarding future treatment options.

Recommendations

1. Schedule a home visit on 11/2/XX to assess current status and, if appropriate, begin weaning the home health aide.
2. Maintain monthly contact with the occupational therapist to assess status and needs.
3. Coordinate disposables cost effectively.
4. Contact account with any change in status.

Diary Date

October 29, 19XX
Sandy Mandell, RN,MA,CRRN,CIRS,CCM
Nurse Case Manager

SAVINGS THIS REPORT PERIOD

Hard Savings

Item/Service	Regular Cost	Negotiated Cost	Savings
Home health aide	$15.00/hr × 4 hrs/day × 7 days/wk = $1806.00/mo	$13.50/hr × 4 hrs/day × 7 days/wk = $1625.40/mo	$180.60/mo
IV Solumedrol	$325.00/day × 5 days = $1625.00	$200.00/day × 5 days = $1000.00	$625.00
Totals	$3,431.00	$2625.40	$805.60

Soft Savings

By providing preventive home care to ensure maintenance of skin integrity, skin graft and hospitalization have been avoided. These translate into approximate savings of $10,000.00

Total savings this report period (hard and soft): $10,805.00
Cost of case management services: $500.00
Net savings: $10,305.00

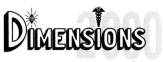

in Managed Care

INSURANCE COMPANY   **February 28, 19XX**

CLIENT   : Sylvia Thompson   **DOL: 19XX**
POLICY #   : 1234567   **DOB: 3/1/XX**
DIMENSIONS # : 148   **SS# : 222-22-2222**

DIAGNOSIS: Multiple Sclerosis

PROGRESS REPORT # 5

Current Status

The client continues to remain at home with home health aide assistance 4 hours per day. She has not had any exacerbation of decubitus. At this time she is able to sit in the chair for up to 7 hours.

The client's status continues to deteriorate. At this time she has lost the use of her right arm and is completely dependent for all activities of daily living. She is unable to propel the wheelchair with the joy stick and now requires installation of a sip-and-puff mechanism. This has been discussed with the account and approved. This case manager has been in contact with the provider, who has been to see the client for a full assessment of wheelchair needs.

With account approval, this case manager met with the provider and the occupational therapist, at the client's home to discuss the needs regarding independence in mobility, in addition to seating accessories to maximize comfort and ensure proper body alignment. The various options were discussed with the client, who stated that she will review the literature describing the differences in adaptive equipment and other accessories. It was decided that within the following week, a definite decision would be made.

On January 5, 19XX, this case manager contacted the client to discuss her choices of accessories. On that same date the provider was contacted to discuss the results of the client's decision and to obtain the cost. The following day the provider faxed to this consultant the cost of all electronic equipment, labor, and miscellaneous charges. The total for a completed chair was quoted at $6,800.00 for the electronic accessories and $3,000.00 for the seating arrangement. This consultant negotiated a cost of $8,500.00 for both. The account was contacted and approved the purchase of the sip-and-puff equipment and the seating equipment at the negotiated rate.

The client was contacted and informed that the chair would be complete and delivered within 3 weeks.

At the time of the home visit this case manager and the occupational therapist discussed the client's increased complaints of spasms and deteriorating musculature. It was recommended that a home physical therapy program might increase the client's comfort and possibly slow the deterioration. This was discussed with the account who approved 4 weeks of home PT. The need for continued therapy would be evaluated after the 4 weeks. The account discussed the benefits language with this case manager and noted that therapy is a covered service, dependent upon rehabilitation potential. The account stated that if therapy is for maintenance only, it is not considered a covered service.

This case manager contacted the physician to discuss the benefits of physical therapy and requested a prescription for a therapist to visit the client at home twice weekly, for 4 weeks, for the purpose of teaching the home health aide and the client's husband proper range of motion exercises. The physician agreed with this consultant's recommendations and faxed a prescription. The therapy provider was then contacted to coordinate care. The cost of therapy was negotiated from $95.00/visit to $80.00/visit.

Summary/Impressions

Although the client continues to deteriorate, she remains motivated to maintain as much independence as possible. She is pleased with the increased independence she will have once the adapted wheelchair is completed.

It is this case manager's opinion that by coordinating short-term physical therapy, the client's comfort level will increase and contracture formation will be avoided through proper range of motion.

It is also this case manager's opinion that continued home health aide assistance at home has prevented complications from decubitus exacerbation.

Recommendations

1. Contact the physical therapist after 3 weeks to assess progress and evaluate for continued need.
2. Contact the client in 3 weeks to ensure receipt of the sip-and-puff wheelchair.
3. Contact the wheelchair provider if any problems with the chair arise and to ensure timely delivery and instruction for use.
4. Contact the account immediately with any changes in status, to discuss further case direction.

Diary Date

March 29, 19XX
Sandy Mandell, RN,MA,CRRN,CIRS,CCM
Nurse Case Manager

SAVINGS

Hard Savings

Item/Service	Regular Cost	Negotiated Cost	Savings
Sip-and-puff wheelchair	$6800.00	$6000.00	$ 800.00
Seating arrangement	$3000.00	$2500.00	$ 500.00
Physical therapy	$95.00/visit × 2/wk × 4 wks = $760.00	$80.00/visit × 2/wk × 4 wks = $640.00	$ 120.00
Totals	$10,560.00	$9140.00	$1420.00

Soft Savings

By maintaining appropriate home care the cost of complications from decubitus exacerbation continue to be avoided. By providing appropriate therapy at home the costly and painful complications from contracture formation will be avoided. Although it is impossible to estimate the cost of quality of life, a minimum of $10,000.00 is saved through avoidance of skin graft surgery and hospitalization (see report dated 9/29/XX).

Total savings this report period: $1420.00
Total savings to date (hard and soft): $14,000.00
Cost of case management to date: $1500.00
Net savings to date: $12,500.00

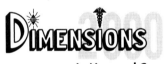

in Managed Care

INSURANCE COMPANY   **July 29, 19XX**

CLIENT   : Sylvia Thompson   **DOL: 19XX**
POLICY #   : 1234567   **DOB: 3/1/XX**
DIMENSIONS # : 148   **SS# : 222-22-2222**

DIAGNOSIS: Multiple Sclerosis

CLOSURE REPORT

Current Status

The client remains medically stable. There has been no further exacerbation of symptoms in the past 3 months. Home health aide assistance has been discontinued. The client can now sit for 8 to 10 hours daily. The skin around the decubitus has toughened and there have been no additional problems in over 1 year.

The client has become proficient with the sip-and-puff wheelchair and is enjoying her mobility independence. She remains optimistic and motivated and is anxious to maintain as much independence as possible.

Range of motion exercises are performed twice daily by the client's husband, who appears to have accepted his wife's disability and limited functional abilities. Through contacts coordinated by this case manager with the MS Society, the client and his wife have gained the appropriate information and knowledge regarding the client's diagnosis and disease process. They have joined a local MS support group and have found comfort in the emotional support offered, in addition to enlarging their social circle.

This case manager contacted the account and discussed this client in depth. It was agreed that at this time further case management services will be discontinued. If the client's status changes this case can be reopened.

Case Summary

This 44-year-old female was diagnosed with multiple sclerosis at the age of 30. She had remained stable and independent until 19X7, when she had to stop working. She remained stable until the spring of 19X3. In September of 19X3, this case manager was contacted to provide on-site case management services.

At that time the client developed a severe sacral decubitus, was deteriorating rapidly, required coordination of home care, and was experiencing increased financial and emotional strain. At that time the client and her husband did not have adequate information regarding the disease process, were hesitant about joining a support group, and appeared overwhelmed with the client's status.

Through case management services this case manager, in collaboration with the account, various providers of care, and the client's physician coordinated appropriate home care to avoid costly complications, arranged for discounted supplies which would be billed directly to the carrier so that the client did not have to lay out the money and wait for reimbursement, coordinated an electronically sophisticated wheelchair to enhance independence, initiated contacts with the MS Society and a local support group, and offered emotional support.

This client has been receiving case management services for 10 months. At this time, since the client is medically stable, no further on-site case management services are needed. This case is now closed.

SAVINGS

Hard Savings

Item/Service	Regular Cost	Negotiated Cost	Savings
Home health aide	$15.00/hr × 4 hr/day × 7 days/wk × 8 mo = $14,448.00	$13.50/hr × 4 hr/day × 7 days/wk × 8 mo = $13,003.20	$ 1444.80
	× 2 hr/day × 5 days/wk × 6 wks = $900.00	× 2 hr/day × 5 days/wk × 6 wks = $810.00	$ 90.00
IV Solumedrol	$1625.00	$1000.00	$ 625.00
Meds/Supplies	$350.00/mo	$275.00/mo	$ 900.00/yr
Therapy	$95.00/visit × 8 = $760.00	$80.00/visit × 8 = $640.00	$ 120.00
Wheelchair & seating	$9800.00	$8500.00	$1300.00
Totals	$27,883.00	$24,228.20	$4479.80/yr

Soft Savings

Appropriate case management services saved a minimum of $10,000.00 through avoidance of skin graft and hospitalization. Additional hospital costs for recurrent pneumonia, estimated at $5000.00, have been avoided through appropriate home care. (The client had a history of four hospitalizations for pneumonia within 2 years. Since case management services have been in place the client has not had any hospitalizations). A cost cannot be placed on the client's increased comfort, increased quality of life, and decreased emotional stress.

Total soft savings: $15,000.00
Total savings (hard and soft): $19,479.80
Total cost case management: $3,000.00
Total net savings: $16,479.80

$5.49 saved for every dollar spent

Sandy Mandell, RN,MA,CRRN,CIRS,CCM
Nurse Case Manager

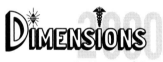

in Managed Care

INSURANCE COMPANY   November 1, 19XX

CLIENT	: **Morris Cohen**	**DOL: 7/1/19XX**
POLICY #	: **891234**	**DOB: 3/1/XX**
DIMENSIONS #	: **149**	**SS# : 222-22-2222**

DIAGNOSIS: Herniated disc (L5-S1)

INITIAL REPORT

History of Loss

On July 1, 19XX, this 43-year-old construction worker was lifting several pieces of sheetrock when he felt "a sharp pain" in his lower back. He states that he immediately felt "a shock-like feeling" shooting down his left leg. He states he was unable to stand up and needed assistance. The client stated that he was taken by ambulance to Central Hospital, New Jersey, where he was treated in the emergency room and discharged to home. The emergency room physician told the client to remain on bed rest for 3 days.

After 3 days the client continued to complain of pain. He called Dr. Hushami, his family physician, who referred him to Dr. Yang, an orthopedic specialist. Dr. Yang examined the client and prescribed physical therapy for 6 weeks.

The client received physical therapy with a therapist who worked in Dr. Yang's office. After 6 weeks the client continued to complain of pain, with minimal improvement. Dr. Yang continued to send the client for physical therapy.

The client has been unable to return to work since the date of injury.

On October 15, 19XX, this client was referred for case management services. On October 17, 19XX this case manager received authorization from the client's attorney to proceed with case management services. The client was contacted by phone and an appointment was scheduled for October 20, 19XX for an initial evaluation to take place at the client's home. The client's wife was present throughout the interview.

This consultant's role was explained to the client and his wife, who both expressed understanding. They both remained cooperative and friendly throughout the interview and answered all questions openly and honestly. The client did not want to sign the consent for medical information until he spoke with his attorney. The consent form was left with the client who stated that he would mail it after he spoke with his attorney.

Current Status

The client continues to complain of pain in the lower back. He states the pain is constant and describes it as "an electric shock running down my leg." He complains of pain in the left groin and down the left leg to his toes. He states that he feels numbness and tingling, however, less than during the first few weeks following the injury. The client states that he has difficulty sleeping at night due to pain. He cannot walk for more than one block and cannot sit comfortably for more than 15 to 20 minutes. He states that the pain is increased when he bends down. He is unable to turn, twist, kneel, or climb stairs. He states that he is unable to lift or carry more than about 5 lb. He also complains of increased pain when he reaches or stretches. He denies bladder or bowel incontinence. It is unknown if he has a problem getting or maintaining an erection, since he states that he has been unable to have sex with his wife since the injury due to pain.

The client stated that his wife assists him every morning with getting dressed and with showering. He is unable to assist with any household chores.

The client appeared to be in significant pain throughout the interview. He frequently shifted his position in the chair. With most movements, facial grimmacing was noted. The client appeared to have difficulty sitting down and rising from the chair.

The client denied having an MRI and stated that the only x-rays that were taken were in the emergency room on the date of injury. He continues to treat with Dr. Yang and continues to receive physical therapy three times per week at the same facility. Therapy includes electrical stimulation, massage, ultrasound, and heat. The client notes minimal improvement in his status since the injury.

Current Medications

Naprosyn: 200 mg twice daily
Inderal: 20 mg daily

Medical History

The client denies any previous workers' compensation injuries. He denies any injuries sustained in a motor vehicle accident.

The client stated a history of colon cancer 3 years ago. He underwent surgery, followed by 6 weeks of radiation. No further treatment was necessary. He reports a 20-year history of hypertension, which has been treated by medication. He reports hernia surgery 15 years ago.

Any other significant medical history was denied.

The client smokes 1 to 1½ packs of cigarettes daily. He states he is "a social drinker." He stated that he usually has a "few beers on weekends" but denies drinking during the week. He denies using or abusing illegal drugs.

Socioeconomic

The client lives in a small, two-bedroom apartment on the second floor of a building without an elevator, in a residential area. He lives with his wife and 9-year-old son. His wife works part-time as a cashier in the local supermarket. She coordinates her work with her son's hours at school.

The client stated that he is having difficulty paying his bills since the injury. He states that he has been using up his savings and has borrowed money from family and friends. The client stated that prior to the injury he was earning almost $50,000.00 per year with overtime. He stated that since the injury he is bringing home $750.00 every 2 weeks. He stated that his rent is $800.00 per month, which leaves little for other expenses. The client stated that he is concerned that he will not be able to maintain his car payments. He stated $2500.00 in credit card debt.

Educational / Vocational Status

The client graduated high school in 19XX. He denies attending vocational school.

He served in the military (Navy) from 19XX to 19XX.

He denies any specific skills.

The client joined the union in 19XX and has worked in construction, through the union hall, for the past 15 years.

The client states that his job duties entail lifting, pushing, and pulling up to 100 lb; climbing ladders; twisting, turning, squatting, bending, walking, standing, and kneeling. He states that there is no light duty available.

Physician

Dr. Yang, orthopedist
111 Main Ave
Anywhere, NJ

201-111-1111

This case manager attempted to contact the physician. His office manager stated that all questions should be forwarded in writing. In addition, the physician will charge $75.00 to respond in writing. The office manager refused to forward progress notes without a signed consent.

Therapist

Joseph Zwyck, physical therapist
address and phone as above

This case manager attempted to contact the therapist on four occasions. To date no return calls have been received.

Employer Contact

This case manager contacted the employer, who stated that the client has been a good employee. He stated that he was anxious to have the client return to work. He stated that there was no light duty available, either permanent or temporary.

The job description given was equivalent to that the client gave.

Summary/Impressions

It is this case manager's opinion that the client is in a significant amount of pain. He appears motivated to return to work. He appeared frustrated and depressed regarding his injury and is fearful for the future regarding his financial ability to support his family.

Dr. Yang appears uncooperative and has refused to supply this case manager with any medical records or information. The therapist, who is located in Dr. Yang's office, has also been uncooperative. It is apparent that the client's current treatment plan has failed to improve his symptoms. It is also apparant that after 3 months of physical therapy, continued therapy will not produce any significant change. This case manager also questions 3 months of therapy that included modalities[3] only. Per the client, he has not had any aggressive therapy.

It is this case manager's opinion that Dr. Wong be contacted to schedule an IME, with takeover treatment. This case manager recommends authorization for an MRI, if Dr. Wong requests.

---

[3]Modalities refer to heat, ultrasound, electrical stimulation and massage. Modalities do not include aggressive physical therapy.

Recommendations

1. With account approval, schedule and attend an IME with takeover treatment with Dr. Wong by 11/15/XX, to assess diagnosis, treatment plan, and time frames.
2. If Dr. Wong recommends an MRI, authorize and schedule as soon as possible.
3. Maintain contact with the client to assess status and progress

Diary Date

December 1, 19XX
Sandy Mandell, RN,MA,CRRN,CIRS,CCM
Nurse Case Manager

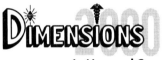

in Managed Care

INSURANCE COMPANY   **December 1, 19XX**

CLIENT   : **Morris Cohen**   **DOL: 7/1/19XX**
POLICY #   : **891234**   **DOB: 3/1/XX**
DIMENSIONS # : **149**   **SS# : 222-22-2222**

DIAGNOSIS: Herniated disc (L5-S1)

PROGRESS REPORT

Current Status

With account approval this case manager scheduled and attended an appointment for the client with Dr. Wong on November 20, 19XX.

Dr. Wong was informed that he would now be the only authorized treating physician. The client was aware.

Dr. Wong examined the client and reviewed all medical records. He requested an MRI of the lumbar spine prior to recommending a treatment plan. This was authorized and scheduled to be done on November 23, 19XX at Medical Imaging. A follow-up appointment was scheduled with Dr. Wong for November 28, 19XX for the purpose of determining the results of the MRI and Dr. Wong's recommended treatment plan.

With account approval the November 28th appointment was attended with the client. Dr. Wong stated that the MRI indicated a herniated disc at level L5-S1. He recommended 6 weeks of aggressive therapy, after which he would determine if surgery were necessary.

The account was contacted to discuss Dr. Wong's recommendations. The account authorized 6 weeks of aggressive therapy. A follow-up appointment with Dr. Wong was scheduled for December 15, 19XX to assess the client's status, improvement, and continued treatment recommendations. Therapy was coordinated at Square Physical Therapy. The cost was negotiated to $85.00/session. The regular cost was $95.00/session.

Summary/Impressions

The client continues to complain of pain. Takeover treatment has been coordinated with Dr. Wong who stated that the client has an L5-S1 herniated disc, directly related to the client's work injury. Prior to surgical intervention Dr. Wong recommended aggressive therapy. Although the client has been going for physical therapy for over 3 months, he has not had any aggressive therapy.

The client stated that he was pleased with Dr. Wong and was optimistic that he would finally be receiving appropriate treatment. The client remains compliant, cooperative and motivated to return to work.

Recommendations

1. Contact the physical therapist during the week of December 10, 19XX to assess client's attendance, compliance, and status.

2. Attend the client's December 15, 19XX appointment with Dr. Wong to assess MMI[4] and return-to-work date, or continuing treatment plan.

Diary Date

January 1, 19XX
Sandy Mandell, RN,MA,CRRN,CIRS,CCM
Nurse Case Manager

---

[4]MMI refers to maximum medical improvement. This term is used with worker's compensation cases to determine when the client can either be released to return to work, or discharged from medical treatment.

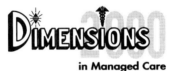

in Managed Care

INSURANCE COMPANY   **April 1, 19XX**

CLIENT	: Morris Cohen	**DOL: 7/1/19XX**
POLICY #	: 891234	**DOB: 3/1/XX**
DIMENSIONS #	: 149	**SS# : 222-22-2222**

DIAGNOSIS: Herniated disc (L5-S1)

CLOSURE REPORT

Current Status

This client was referred for case management services on October 15, 19XX. This 43-year-old construction worker sustained a herniated disc at L5-S1 in a work-related accident. He treated with Dr. Yang, who prescribed physical therapy. After 3 months the client continued to complain of pain, with little improvement noted.

Takeover treatment was coordinated with Dr. Wong, November 19XX. An MRI was authorized, which documented a herniated disc. Dr. Wong recommended aggressive physical therapy, three times per week, for 6 weeks. After 6 weeks of aggressive therapy, the client noted significant improvement. Dr. Wong recommended 6 more weeks of therapy at a work-hardening facility.[5]

On February 15, 19XX, the client no longer complained of radiating pain down his leg. He stated an increased level of activity, with only occasional back pain. Dr. Wong released the client to return to work as of March 1, 19XX.

On March 5, 19XX, the client was contacted. He stated that he did return to work on March 1st and was able to perform his job duties, with only occasional periods of discomfort.

Since the client returned to work and has been discharged from medical care, this case is now closed.

Sandy Mandell, RN,MA,CRRN,CIRS,CCM
Nurse Case Manager

COST SAVINGS

Hard savings: Physical therapy—$15.00/visit × 18 = $270.00

Soft savings: Had the client continued treating with Dr. Yang, he might have continued with therapy for approximately 3 more months (three times per week). The therapist at Dr. Yang's office was charging $95.00 per visit. Savings over three months = $3,420.00. Without case management services it is doubtful that the client would have been able to return to work by March 1, 19XX. Savings of additional 3 months' benefits = $4,500.00

Total savings (soft and hard): $8190.00

Cost of case management services: $1500.00

Net savings: $6690.00

---

[5] Work hardening is a form of physical therapy which simulates job duties that the client must perform.

Resources II

AIDS/HIV

- AIDS Research Information   (410) 342-2742
  Center, Inc. (ARIC)   e-mail: aricinc@Clark.net
  20 South Ellwood Avenue, Suite 2
  Baltimore, MD 21224-2241
  research, information

- AIDS Treatment Data Network   (800) 734-7104
  611 Broadway   e-mail: AIDSTreatD@aol.com
  Suite 613
  New York, NY 10012-2608
  treatment information

- American Foundation for AIDS Research   (800) 392-6327
  733 Third Avenue, 12th Floor
  New York, NY 10017
  research, education

- Centers for Disease Control (CDC)   (404) 377-9563
  Center for Infectious Diseases
  1600 Clifton Road
  Atlanta, GA 30333
  information, research, education, policy formation

- Gay Men's Health Crisis   (212) 807-6664
    129 West 20th Street
    New York, NY 10011
        information, education

- God's Love, We Deliver   (212) 294-8100
    166 Avenue of the Americas
    New York, NY 10013-1207
        food delivery, NY area only

- Kaposi's Sarcoma Research and Education   (415) 864-4376
    470 Castro Street, #207
    PO Box 3360
    San Francisco, CA 94114
        research, education for Kaposi's sarcoma

- Mothers of AIDS Patients   (619) 234-3432
    3403 East Street
    San Diego, CA 92101
        support, information

- National AIDS Information   (800) 342-AIDS (English)
    Clearing House   (800) 344-SIDA (Spanish)
    PO Box 6003
    Rockville, MD 20850
        information, material

- National Association of People with AIDS   (202) 898-0414
    1413 K Street NW, 7th Floor
    Washington, DC 20005
        support, education, information

- National Pediatric and Family HIV   (800) 362-0071
    Resource Center
    15 S 9 Street
    Newark, NJ 07107
        information

- NY State Department of Health
    AIDS Drug Assistance Program (ADAP)
    ADAP plus
        financial assistance

- People with AIDS Coalition (PWA)   (212) 627-1810
  236A West 19th Street, #125
  New York, NY 10011
      information, support

- Project Inform   (415) 558-8669
  1965 Market Street, Suite 220
  San Francisco, CA 94103
      treatment information

- Ryan White National Fund   (800) 933-KIDS
  c/o Athletes and Entertainers for Kids
  PO Box 191, Building B
  Gardens, CA 90248
      services, information

- San Francisco AIDS Foundation   (415) 864-4376
  333 Valencia Street, 4th floor
  PO Box 6182
  San Francisco, CA 94101-6182
      education, referrals for assistance with social security,
      housing, legal, and medical needs

- Shanti Project   (415) 558-9644
  890 Hayes Street
  San Francisco, CA 94117
      counseling, support

- Social Security Administration   (301) 594-1234
  6401 Security Boulevard
  Baltimore, MD 21235
      funds Medicare programs

- State AIDS Policy Center
  Intergovernmental Health Policy Center
  2011 I Street NW, Suite 200
  Washington, DC 20006
      information, policy formation

- World Health Organization (WHO)   (404) 239-3311
  Collaborating Center on AIDS
  c/o Centers for Disease Control
  1600 Clifton Road, NE
  Atlanta, GA 30333
       educational materials

CANCER

- American Cancer Society   (800) 227-2345
  National Office
  90 Park Avenue
  New York, NY 10016
       research, information

- Cancer Care, Inc.   (212) 679-5700
  1 Park Avenue
  New York, NY 10016
       social work assistance, bereavement counseling,
       financial assistance

- Candlelighters Foundation   (202) 659-5136
  2025 I Street NW
  Washington, DC 20006
       self-help for parents of children or adolescents with cancer

- Hospice Educational Institute   (203) 767-1620
  PO Box 713
  5 Essex Square, Suite 3B
  Essex, CT 06426
       public and professional information

- Leukemia Society of America, Inc.   (703) 960-1100
  2900 Eisenhower Avenue #419
  Alexandria, VA 22314
       information

- National Hospice Organization   (703) 243-5900
  1901 Fort Meyer Drive, Suite 402
  Arlington, VA 22209
       information

- National Cancer Cytology Center   (516) 349-0610
  88 Sunnyside Boulevard, Suite 204
  Plainview, NY 11803
  information on cancer screening

- Reach to Recovery   (212) 973-8759
  90 Park Avenue
  New York, NY 10016
  support group for victims of breast cancer

- United Cancer Council, Inc.   (317) 923-6490
  1803 N. Meridian Street, Room 202
  Indianapolis, IN 46202
  research, information

- United Ostomy Association   (213) 255-4681
  1111 Wilshire Boulevard
  Los Angeles, CA 90017
  support, information

CARDIOVASCULAR DISEASE

- American Heart Association   (214) 373-6300
  72–72 Greenville Avenue
  Dallas, TX 75231
  research, information

- National Hypertension Association   (212) 889-3557
  324 East 30th Street
  New York, NY 10016
  information, education

CHILDBIRTH

- Childbirth Education Foundation   (215) 357-2792
  PO Box 5
  Richboro, PA 18954

- La Leche League International
  9616 Minneapolis Avenue
  PO Box 1209
  Franklin Park, IL 60131
    assistance for breast feeding mothers,
    seminars, information

- Planned Parenthood Federation of America   (800) 829-7732
  810 Seventh Avenue   (212) 541-7800
  New York, NY 10019
    information, sex education

CHILDREN

- American Juvenile Arthritis Organization   (404) 872-7110
  1314 Spring Street
  Atlanta, GA 30309
    advocacy for children with arthritis

- Association for Insulin Dependent Diabetes   (212) 889-7575
  c/o Juvenile Diabetes Foundation International
  60 Madison Avenue
  New York, NY 10010
    self-help, education, workshops

- Association of Birth Defects in Children   (407) 245-7035
  3526 Emery Wood Lane
  Orlando, FL 32806
    information, statistics, research

- Association of Maternal Child   (202) 775-0436
  Health Programs
  1350 Connecticut Avenue NW, Suite 803
  Washington, DC 20036
    research, education

- Association of Retarded Citizens   (817) 640-0204
  PO Box 6109
  Arlington, TX 76005
    advocacy, education

- Autism Society of America   (800) 3-AUTISM
    7910 Woodmont Avenue, Suite 650   (301) 657-0881
    Bethesda, MD 20814
        education, information

- Children's Hospice International   (703) 684-4464
    1800 Diagonal Road, Suite 600
    Alexandria, VA 22314
        information

- Children's Liver Foundation   (201) 761-1111
    28 Highland Avenue
    Maplewood, NJ 07040
        research, support, information

- Children's Lung Association of America   (404) 993-5859
    150 Pond Way
    Roswell, GA 30076
        research, education

- Cystic Fibrosis Foundation   (301) 951-4422
    6931 Arlington Road
    Bethesda, MD 20814
        research, family assistance

- Human Growth Foundation   (612) 831-2780
    4930 West 77th Street, Suite 150
    Minneapolis, MN 55435
        research, education on growth disorders

- Juvenile Diabetes Association   (212) 889-7575
    23 East 26th Street
    New York, NY 10010
        research, information

- March of Dimes Birth Defects Foundation   (914) 428-7100
    1275 Mamaroneck Avenue
    White Plains, NY 10605
        research, information

- Mental Retardation Association   (801) 328-1575
    211 E. 300 South Street, Suite 212
    Salt Lake City, UT 84111
        advocacy, research, education

- Muscular Dystrophy Association   (520) 529-2000
    3300 E. Sunrise Drive
    Tucson, AZ 85718
        research, information

- National Association for Downs Syndrome   (312) 543-6060
    PO Box 63
    Oak Park, IL 60303
        parental support

- National Association for Sickle Cell   (800) 421-8453
    Disease, Inc.   (213) 736-5455
    3345 Wilshire Boulevard, Suite 1106
    Los Angeles, CA 90010
        research, information

- National Association of Retarded Citizens   (817) 261-4961
    2501 Avenue J
    Arlington, TX 76011
        political advocacy

- National Center for Education Materials and   (614) 422-7596
    Medica for the Handicapped
    Ohio State University
    Faculty for Exceptional Children
    Columbus, OH 43210
        information, education

- National Hemophilia Foundation   (212) 219-8180
    10 Greene Street, Suite 303
    New York, NY 10012
        research, information

- National Parent Network on Disabilities
    1600 Prince Street, #115
    Alexandria, VA 22314
        information, support

- Shriner's Hospital for Crippled Children   (813) 885-2575
    PO Box 25356
    Tampa, FL 33622
        assistance in care of handicapped children

- The Association for the Severely   (206) 283-5055
  Handicapped
    1600 West Amory Way
    Seattle, WA 98119
        information, support

- United Cerebral Palsy Association, Inc.   (202) 842-1266
    1660 L Street NW, Suite 700
    Washington, DC 20036
        information

- United Way Resource Center   (619) 492-2115
    PO Box 23543
    San Diego, CA 92123
        support, referral information

DIABETES

- American Diabetes Association   (703) 549-1500
    National Service Center   (800) 232-3472
    PO Box 25757
    1660 Duke Street
    Alexandria, VA 22313
        research, information, education

- Becton Dickenson   (800) 627-1579
    Consumer Products
    Franklin Lakes, NJ 07417
        materials for client education

- Joslin Diabetes Center   (617) 732-2415
    Joslin Place
    Boston, MA 02215
        information, education, program for diabetes control

- Juvenile Diabetes Association   (212) 889-7575
    23 East 26th Street
    New York, NY 10010
        research, public information

- National Diabetes Information   (301) 468-2162
  Clearinghouse
  Box NDIC
  Bethesda, MD 20892
  information

FINANCIAL ASSISTANCE

- Catastrophic Illness in Children Relief   (800) 335-FUND
  Fund Commission
  CN 700
  Trenton, NJ 08625
  financial assistance for parents with
  catastrophically ill children

- Health Care Financing Administration   (202) 245-6726
  200 Independence Avenue SW
  Washington, DC 20201
  funds federal health programs

- Social Security Administration   (301) 594-3120
  6401 Security Building
  Baltimore, MD 21235
  administers Medicare programs

- World Medical Relief   (313) 866-5333
  11745 Rosa Parks Boulevard
  Detroit, MI 48206

GERIATRICS

- Alzheimer's Disease & Related   (312) 853-3060
  Disorders Association
  70 East Lake Street
  Chicago, IL 60601
  research, education, support

- American Association of Retired Persons   (800) 293-3900
  3200 E. Corson Street
  Lakewood, CA 90712
     advocacy, cooperative buying programs
     for insurance and medications

- American Society on Aging   (415) 543-2617
  833 Market Street
  San Francisco, CA 94103
     advocacy, legislation, information

- Gerontological Society   (202) 466-6750
  1835 K Street NW, Suite 305
  Washington, DC 20006
     research

- National Council on Aging   (202) 479-1200
  409 3rd Street SW
  Washington, DC 20024
     information

- National Geriatrics Society   (414) 272-4130
  212 W. Wisconsin Avenue
  Milwaukee, WI 53203
     research, education

- National Institute on Aging   (301) 496-4000
  9000 Rockville Pike, Building 31   (301) 496-9265
  Bethesda, MD 20892
     research

HEALTH PROMOTION

- Action on Smoking & Health   (202) 659-4310
  2013 H Street NW
  Washington, DC 20006
     public advocacy

- American College of Preventive Medicine
  1015 15 Street NW, Suite 403
  Washington, DC 20005
     information on health promotion programs

- American Health Foundation
  320 East 43rd Street
  New York, NY 10018
    information, research

- American Hospital Association
  840 North Lake Shore Drive
  Chicago, IL 60611
    health promotion literature

- A Wellness Center, Inc.   (212) 532-4286
  15 East 40th Street, Suite 704
  New York, NY 10016
    information, education

- Do It Now Foundation   (602) 257-0797
  PO Box 21126
  Phoenix, AZ 85036
    self-help, information

- Healthy America
  315 West 105th Street, #1F
  New York, NY 10025
    advocacy, information

- U.S. Department of Health and Human Services
  Office of Health Education and Health Promotion
  Washington, DC 20203
    information for health education

- Wellness Association   (707) 632-5398
  5433–E
  Mill Valley, CA 94942
    education, resources to improve health

HEARING IMPAIRED

- Alexander Graham Bell Association   (202) 337-5220
  for the Deaf
  3417 Volta Place NW
  Washington, DC 20007
    advocacy, information

- American Speech–Language–   (301) 897-5700
  Hearing Association
  10801 Rockville Pike
  Rockville, MD 20852
  research, information

- Better Hearing Institute   (703) 642-0580
  PO Box 1840
  Washington, DC 20013
  information

- Deafness Research Foundation   (212) 684-6556
  55 East 34th Street
  New York, NY 10016
  education, research, sponsors National Temporal Bone Bank

- Hearing Industries Association   (202) 833-1411
  1800 M Street NW
  Washington, DC 20036
  research, information

- National Association of the Deaf   (301) 587-1788
  814 Thayer Avenue
  Silver Spring, MD 20910
  advocacy, education, legislation

- Telecommunications for the Deaf   (301) 589-3786
  8719 Colesville Road, #300
  Silver Spring, MD 20910
  information

HOSPICE

- Children's Hospice International   (703) 684-4464
  1800 Diagonal Road, Suite 600
  Alexandria, VA 22314
  information

- Hospice Educational Institute   (203) 767-1620
  PO Box 713
  5 Essex Square, Suite 3B
  Essex, CT 06426
  information

- National Hospice Organization   (703) 243-5900
  1901 Ft. Meyer Drive, Suite 402
  Arlington, VA 22209
  information

LUNG

- American Lung Association   (212) 315-8700
  1740 Broadway
  New York, NY 10019
  research, information, education

- Emphysema Anonymous, Inc.   (813) 334-4226
  PO Box 66
  Ft. Meyers, FL 33902
  self-help

- National Asthma Center
  875 Avenue of the Americas
  New York, NY
  information

- National Foundation for Asthma, Inc.   (602) 624-7481
  PO Box 50304
  Tucson, AZ 85703
  outpatient treatment

- National Jewish Center for Immunology   (800) 573-5864
  and Respiratory Medicine
  1400 Jackson Street
  Denver, CO 80206
  information, research

MENTAL HEALTH

- American Academy of Child and   (202) 966-7300
  Adolescent Psychiatry
  3615 Wisconsin Avenue NW
  Washington, DC 20016
  research

- American Association of Psychiatric Services   (202) 659-9115
  for Children
    1725 K Street NW, Suite 1112
    Washington, DC 20006
        referral for child counseling

- American Institute of Stress   (914) 963-1200
    124 Park Avenue
    Yonkers, NY 10703
        information, education

- Hogg Foundation for Mental Health
    University of Texas, Austin
    PO Box 7998
    University Station
    Austin, TX 78712
        information

- National Clearinghouse for Mental Health
    National Institute of Mental Health
    Room 11A33, Parklawn Building
    5600 Fishers Lane
    Rockville, MD 20857
        information, education

- National Consortium for   (202) 462-3755
  Child Mental Health Services
    1424 16th Street NW, Suite 201A
    Washington, DC 20036
        information

- National Council of   (301) 984-6200
  Community Mental Health Centers
    6101 Montrose Road, Suite 360
    Rockville, MD 20285
        information

- National Mental Health Association   (703) 684-7722
    1021 Prince Street
    Arlington, VA 22314
        advocates for the mentally ill

NEUROMUSCULAR PROBLEMS

- American Paralysis Association   (800) 225-0292
  500 Morris Avenue
  Springfield, NJ 07081
  information, materials

- Amyotrophic Lateral Sclerosis Society   (800) 782-4747
  of America
  21021 Ventura Boulevard, Suite 321
  Woodland Hills, CA 91364
  information

- Huntington's Disease Society of America
  140 West 22nd Street, 6th floor
  New York, NY 10011-2420
  research, information

- Miami Project   (305) 243-6001
  1600 NW 10th Avenue, Room 48
  Miami, FL 33136
  research

- National Multiple Sclerosis Society   (212) 986-3240
  733 Third Avenue, 6th floor
  New York, NY 10017
  information, research

- National Spinal Cord Injury Foundation   (617) 935-2722
  600 W. Cummings Park, Suite 2000   (800) 962-9629
  Woburn, MA 01801
  information, statistics

- Paralyzed Veterans of America   (202) 245-7246
  4350 East West Highway, Suite 900
  Washington, DC 20014
  information, support

- Petrofsky Center for Rehabilitation   (714) 855-4837
  and Research
  13765 Alton Parkway, Suite E
  Irvine, CA 92718

- Society for the Advancement of Travel
  for the Handicapped
  327 Fifth Avenue, Suite 610
  New York, NY 10016
  information about travel

- The System-Accessible Design and Product
  Information System from Information
  Development Corp.
  360 St. Albin Court
  Winston Salem, NC 27104
  information

PAIN MANAGEMENT

- National Chronic Pain Outreach   (703) 368-7357
  8222 Wycliffe Ct.
  Manassas, VA 22110
  information, support

- National Commission on the Treatment   (301) 983-1710
  of Intractable Pain
  PO Box 9553, Friendship Station
  Washington, DC 20016
  information, assistance

- Traditional Acupuncture Institute   (301) 596-6006
  American City Building, Suite 100
  Columbia, MD 21044
  education, legal information

SUBSTANCE ABUSE

- Al-Anon Family Group Headquarters   (212) 481-6565
  PO Box 182
  Madison Square Station
  New York, NY 10159
  self-help recovery for family members of alcoholics

- Alcohol Research Information Service   (517) 485-9900
  1106 East Oakland
  Lansing, MI 48906
  teaching material, information, statistics

- Alcoholics Anonymous World Services   (212) 686-1100
  PO Box 459
  Grand Central Station
  New York, NY 10163
      recovery program, chapters nationwide

- American Council for Drug Education   (301) 984-5700
  5820 Hubbard Drive
  Rockville, MD 20852
      information, research

- American Council on Alcohol Problems   (314) 739-5944
  3426 Bridgeland Drive
  Bridgeton, MO 63044
      research, information, education, legislation

- Alcohol, Drug Abuse and   (301) 443-4797
  Mental Health Administration
  5600 Fishers Lane
  Baltimore, MD 20857
      research, information

- International Council for Prevention   (202) 722-6729
  of Alcoholism and Drug Dependency
  6830 Laurel Street NW
  Washington, DC 20012
      research, information

- National Institute on Alcohol Abuse   (301) 443-3885
  and Alcoholism
  5600 Fishers Lane
  Baltimore, MD 20857
      research, information, rehabilitation training

VIOLENCE/CHILD ABUSE/RAPE

- Batterers Anonymous   (714) 355-1100
  1269 North E Street
  San Bernardino, CA 92405
      self-help group for male abusers

- Emerge   (617) 547-9870
    18 Hurley Street, Suite 23
    Cambridge, MA 02141
        counseling for men for prevention of abuse
- Feminist Alliance Against Rape   (202) 686-9463
    PO Box 21033
    Washington, DC 20009
        education, self-defense
- National Coalition Against Domestic Violence   (202) 638-6388
    PO Box 34103   (800) 333-SAFE
    Washington, DC 20043-4103
        safe haven information
- National Council on Child Abuse &   (202) 429-6695
  Family Violence
    1050 Connecticut Avenue NW, Suite 300
    Washington, DC 20036
        education
- Rape Crisis Center
    PO Box 21005
    Washington, DC 20009
        information for victims of rape

VISUAL IMPAIRMENT

- American Council of the Blind   (800) 424-8666
    1155 Vermont Avenue NW, Suite 720
    Washington, DC 20005
        information
- American Foundation for the Blind, Inc.   (800) 232-5463
    15 West 16th Street
    New York, NY 10011
        information, workshops, seminars
- Association for Education and Rehabilitation
  of the Blind and Visually Impaired
    206 N. Washington Street, Suite 320
    Alexandria, VA 22314
        information, education

- Braille Institute   (213) 663-1111
  741 Vermont Avenue
  Los Angeles, CA 90029
      training in Braille

- Carroll Center for the Blind   (612) 969-6200
  770 Centre Street
  Newton, MA 02158
      rehabilitation and training for the blind

- Christian Record Braille Foundation, Inc.   (402) 488-0981
  PO Box 6097
  Lincoln, NE 68506
      Braille and large-type books and magazines—free; cassettes

- Eye Bank for Sight Restoration, Inc.   (212) 980-6700
  210 East 64th Street   (212) 838-9211
  New York, NY 10021
      provides donor tissue for corneal transplants

- Guide Dog Foundation for the Blind   (800) 548-4337
  371 E. Jericho Turnpike
  Smithtown, NY 11787
      trains dogs for the blind

- Leader Dogs for the Blind   (313) 651-9011
  1039 Rochester Road
  Rochester, MI 48063
      trains dogs for the blind

- Local Lions Clubs
      provide eye glasses

- National Association for Visually Handicapped   (212) 889-3141
  305 East 24th Street
  New York, NY 10010
      counseling, books, information

- National Society to Prevent Blindness   (800) 221-3004
  National Center for Sight
  500 E. Remington Road
  Schaumburg, IL 60173
      information, education

OTHER

- American Burn Association
  c/o Shriners Burns Institute
  202 Goodman Street
  Cincinnati, OH 45219
  information

- American Coalition of   (202) 785-4265
  Citizens with Disabilities (ACCD)
  1200 15th Street NW, Suite 201
  Washington, DC 20005
  advocacy, information

- American Juvenile Arthritis Organization   (404) 872-7110
  1314 Spring Street
  Atlanta, GA 30309
  advocacy for children with arthritis

- American Liver Association
  998 Pomton Avenue
  Cedar Grove, NJ 07009
  research, information

- American Lupus Society Information
  260 Maple Court, Suite 123
  Ventura, CA 93003
  information

- American Parkinson Disease Association   (800) 223-2732
  60 Bay Street, Suite 401
  Staten Island, NY 18901
  information

- American Red Cross
  17th and D Streets NW
  Washington, DC 20006
  disaster assistance, information

- Arthritis Foundation   (404) 872-7100
  PO Box 19000   (800) 283-7800
  Atlanta, GA 30326
  information

- Arthritis Rehabilitation Center   (202) 223-5320
  1234 19th Street NW
  Washington, DC 20036
       diagnostic and treatment services

- Arthritis Society   (416) 967-1414
  920 Young Street, Suite 420
  Toronto, Canada M4W 3J7
       research, information

- Association for Vital Records and Health Statistics
  c/o George vanAmburg
  Michigan Department of Public Health
  3423 Logan Street, North
  PO Box 30195
  Lansing, MI 48909
       *The only national forum for study and discussion of solutions
       of health care problems related to vital statistics*

- *Case Management Resource Guide*   (800) 627-2244
  Center for Consumer Healthcare Information
  PO Box 16067
  Irvine, CA 92713
       *A resource guide for the practicing case manager. Updated
       yearly, the 4-volume guide includes the following categories:
       home care, rehabilitation services, psychiatric treatment pro-
       grams, addiction treatment programs, nursing facilities, and
       adult day care*

- Disability Rights Center   (202) 223-3304
  1346 Connecticut Avenue NW, Suite 1124
  Washington, DC 20036
       information

- Easter Seal Society for Crippled Children and Adults
  2023 W. Ogden Avenue
  Chicago, IL 60612
       research, information, assistance

- Epilepsy Foundation of America   (301) 459-3700
  4351 Garden City Drive
  Landover, MD 20785
       research, information

- Health Insurance Association of America   (800) 828-0111
  555 13th Street NW, Suite 600 E
  Washington, DC 20004
  information, statistics

- Health Resources and Services Administration   (301) 443-2086
  5600 Fishers Lane
  Rockville, MD 20857
  information

- Hepatitis Foundation International
  Box 222
  Cedar Grove, NJ 07009
  information

- Insurance Information Institute   (212) 669-9203
  110 William Street
  New York, NY 10038
  insurance information, statistics

- Integrated Technologies   (908) 221-0926
  PO Box 159
  Basking Ridge, NJ 07920
  environmental control systems

- Joint Commission on Accreditation   (708) 916-5118
  of Health Care Organizations (JCAHO)
  information

- Myasthenia Gravis Foundation   (800) 541-5454
  53 W. Jackson Boulevard, Suite 660
  Chicago, IL 60604
  research, information

- National Association for Home Care   (202) 547-7424
  519 C Street NE
  Washington, DC 20002
  information

- National Association of Rehabilitation Facilities   (703) 648-9300
  1910 Association Drive, #200
  Reston, VA 22091
  information

- National Council on the Handicapped   (202) 732-1276
  330 C Street SW, Room 3123
  Washington, DC 20202
    information

- National Easter Seal Society   (800) 221-6827
  70 East Lake Street
  Chicago, IL 60601

- National Foundation for Ileitis and Colitis   (800) 343-3637
  444 Park Avenue South
  New York, NY 10018
    research, information

- National Head Injury Foundation   (202) 296-6443
  1776 Massachusetts Avenue NW, Suite 100   (800) 444-6443
  Washington, DC 20036
    information, statistics

- National Institute of   (800) 356-4674
  Occupational Safety and Health
  200 Independence Avenue SW
  Washington, DC 20036
    information

- National Institutes of Health   (301) 496-4000
  900 Rockville Pike
  Bethesda, MD 20205
    information

- National Kidney Foundation   (800) 622-9010
  30 East 33rd Street
  New York, NY 10016
    information

- National Organization of Rare Diseases   (800) 999-NORD
  PO Box 8923   (203) 746-6518
  New Fairfield, CT 06812
    information, statistics

- National Rehabilitation Information Center   (800) 346-2742
  8455 Colesville Road, Suite 935
  Silver Spring, MD 20910
    information

- Parkinson's Disease Foundation   (800) 457-6676
    William Black Medical Research Building
    650 W. 168th Street
    New York, NY 10032
        information

- Self Help Center   (800) 336-0341
    Riverwood Center
    PO Box 547
    Benton Harbor, MI 49022
        self-help, support

- W.K. Kellog Foundation
    400 North Avenue
    Battle Creek, MI 49017
        information, grants

HOTLINES

- AIDS   (800) 342-AIDS
- Alcoholism   (800) 328-9000
- Alzheimer's Disease and Senile Dementia   (800) 621-0379
- Asthma and Lung   (800) 222-LUNG
- Cancer   (800) 4-CANCER
- Children's Diseases   (800) 237-5055
- Cystic Fibrosis   (800) FIGHT-CF
- Diabetes   (800) 232-3472
- Down's Syndrome   (800) 221-4602
- Domestic Violence   (800) 333-SAFE
- Drug Abuse   (800) 662-HELP
- General Health Information   (800) 336-4797
- American Heart Association   (800) 634-1242
- Kidney   (800) 638-8299
- Lupus   (800) 558-0121
- Multiple Sclerosis   (800) FIGHT-MS

- Spinal Cord Injury   (800) 526-3456
- SIDS (Sudden Infant Death Syndrome)   (800) 221-SIDS

INTERNET

- Centers for Disease Control
  and Prevention   http://www.cdc.gov
- Department of Health
  and Human Services   http://www.os.dhhs.gov
- Galaxy   http://galaxy.einet.net/galaxy/Medicine.html
- Global Health Network
           http://www.pitt.edu/HOME/GHNet/GHNet.html
- Group Health Cooperative   http://www.ghc.org
- Health Administration Resources
       http://www.mercer.peachnet.edu/www/health/health.html
- Health Care Financing Administration (HCFA)
              http://www.ssa.gov/hcfa/hcfahp2.html
- House of Representatives
              http://www.pls.com:8001/his/usc.html
- Infoseek   http://www.infoseek.com/TBITS/
- Institute of HeartMath
        http://www.webcom.com/-hrtmath/IHM/AboutIHM.html
- JCAHO Survey Reports Archive
            http://www.nnim.nim.nih.gov/nnlm/jcahorep.html
- Martindale's Health Science Guide
             http://sci.lib.uci.edu/~martindale/HSGuide.html
- Medical Matrix
                   http://kuhttp.cc.ukans.edu/cwis/units/
                   medcntr/Lee/HOMEPAGE.html
- MedWeb (electronic newsletters and journals)
             http://www.shadow.net/-arb/medweb.html

- National Committee for Quality Assurance (NCQA)
  http://www.ncqa.org

- National Health Information Center   http://nhicnt.health.org

- National Jewish Center for Immunology
  and Respiratory Medicine   http://www.njc.org

- National Network of Libraries of Medicine
  http://www.nnim.nim.nih.gov/index.html

- Put Prevention Into Practice   http://www.os.dhhs.gov.81/PPIP/

- The Medical Index   http://sledgehammer.camtech.com.au/
  webcomnet/mindex.html

- The Virtual Medical Center
  http://www-sci.lib.uci.edu/martindale/MedicalResources.html

- Webcrawler   http://www.webcrawler.com/

- Yahoo   http://www.com/Health/

Case Management *Certification*

This appendix includes information about several certifications available for case managers.

The following is an appendix outline:

A. Certified case manager (CCM)
   1. Eligibility criteria
   2. Exam categories
   3. Maintaining certification
B. Certified rehabilitation registered nurse (CRRN)
   1. Eligibility criteria
   2. Exam categories
   3. Maintaining certification
C. Certified insurance rehabilitation specialist (CIRS)
   1. Eligibility criteria
   2. Exam categories
   3. Maintaining certification

CERTIFIED CASE MANAGER (CCM)

In February 1992, the Certification of Insurance Rehabilitation Specialist Commission was selected by the National Task Force to develop the process for case management certification. In May

1993, the first CCM exam was given. Given twice yearly, it has quickly become the universal standard to ensure adequate education and experience for the practice of case management.

Eligibility Requirements

Professions of varied backgrounds may be eligible to take the CCM exam. All applicants must hold a license or certification based on a "minimum educational requirement of a post-secondary program in a field that promotes the physical, psychosocial, or vocational well being of the persons being served."[1]

The applicant is required to qualify for one of three categories of employment experience. The categories are differentiated by the length of employment and clinical experience. All categories require experience that reflects direct contact with clients receiving case management. The commission requires that the description of case management services include the following six components: (1) assessment, (2) planning, (3) implementation, (4) coordination, (5) monitoring, and (6) evaluation.

Employment must be verified by the employer, with dates of employment and a written job description.

Exam Categories

The exam consists of 300 multiple-choice questions based on the following five content areas:

1. *Coordination and service delivery.* Includes topics ranging from confidentiality issues through communication of treatment goals.

---

[1]Commission for Case Manager Certification. (1996). CCM certification guide, p. 3.

2. *Physical and psychological factors.* Questions dealing with the ability to identify physical and psychological characteristics of disabling conditions and appropriate resources and treatment protocols.
3. *Benefit systems and cost-benefit analysis.* Includes topics about evaluating and negotiating provider costs.
4. *Case management concepts.* Questions regarding strategies used when providing case management services.
5. *Community resources.* Includes topics about federal legislation, such as the Americans with Disabilities Act; vocational services; adaptive equipment and establishing client support systems.

Maintaining Certification

Upon obtaining a passing score, the case manager receives documentation of certification. The initial certification is valid for 5 years. Certification is renewable every 5 years through continuing professional development. CEUs are available at many seminars and conferences held throughout the year.

For complete details contact:

> The Commission for Case Manager Certification
> 1835 Rohlwing Road, Suite D
> Rolling Meadows, Illinois 60008
> (847) 818-0292

CERTIFIED REHABILITATION REGISTERED NURSE (CRRN)

The Rehabilitation Nursing Certification Board (RNCB) is a component of the Association of Rehabilitation Nurses (ARN), which administers CRRN certification. The first exam was given on

December 7, 1984. Today there are more than 11,000 certified rehabilitation nurses. The exam is given twice yearly.

Eligibility Requirements

Applicants must hold a valid, current RN license. The applicant must also have completed a minimum of 2 years of practice as a registered nurse in the field of rehabilitation within the past 5 years. Employment experience must be validated by two professional colleagues. Rehabilitation nursing employment includes direct patient care, research, and/or the supervision of other persons to achieve or assist in the achievement of the client's goals. As of December 2000, in addition to the existing criteria, a BSN degree will be required, as well as completion of education in the specialty of rehabilitation nursing within 5 years of application.

Exam Categories

The exam consists of 250 multiple-choice questions, divided into five general categories. The categories are: (1) theoretical background, (2) data collection, (3) nursing diagnosis and interventions, (4) purpose and functions of the rehabilitation team, and (5) reintegration of the client into the community.

Maintaining Certification

The initial certification is valid for 5 years. Renewal is based on accumulating continuing education units through seminars, conferences, and/or other educational means.

For complete details contact:

Rehabilitation Nursing Certification Board
5700 Old Orchard Road, first floor
Skokie, IL 60077-1024
(708) 966-3433

CERTIFIED INSURANCE
REHABILITATION SPECIALIST (CIRS)

The Certification of Insurance Rehabilitation Specialists Commission (CIRSC) developed a credentialing process for registered nurses and certified rehabilitation counselors who work in the area of rehabilitation that encompasses services frequently mandated under state insurance laws and government disability programs. Such programs include workers' compensation, personal injury liability, no-fault automobile insurance, longshore and harbor workers' compensation, and social security disability insurance.

The certification exam is administered twice yearly.

Eligibility Requirements

There are four categories of eligibility; the applicant must meet the requirements in one category. The first category requires current, valid licensure as either a registered nurse (RN) or a certified rehabilitation counselor (CRC), with a minimum of 24 months of acceptable employment. The applicant with a masters or doctorate degree may be eligible depending upon course requirements and a minimum of 24 months acceptable employment, as outlined in the CIRS certification guide. The second and third categories set eligibility criteria based on the applicant's educational level (bachelors, with a major in rehabilitation, masters, or doctorate) and course requirements and a minimum of 36 months of acceptable employment. The fourth category outlines criteria for the applicant with a bachelors, masters, or doctorate in any discipline and a minimum of 60 months acceptable employment.

All employment must be verified by employers, including dates of employment and job descriptions.

Exam Categories

The exam is comprised of 300 multiple-choice questions. The exam content is based on five general subject areas as follows:

1. *Job placement and vocational assessment.* Questions cover areas such as conducting labor market surveys, using results of vocational/psychometric evaluations, conducting transferable skills and job-ready analyses, knowledge of labor market information and other issues concerned with employment opportunities for people with disabling conditions.
2. *Case management and human disabilities.* Questions about the nature of various disabling conditions and personality/motivational issues as they relate to the insurance process.
3. *Rehabilitation services and care.* Includes topics dealing with knowledge about available services in the community for the disabled population.
4. *Disability legislation.* Questions about disability legislation and their interrelationships including such areas as the Equal Employment Opportunity Act, Americans with Disabilities Act, Fair Labor Standards Act, Occupational Health and Safety Act, labor union practices, and affirmative action requirements.
5. *Forensic rehabilitation.* Includes topics about courtroom and/or deposition protocols.

Maintaining Certification

The initial certification is valid for 5 years. Renewal is based on accumulating continuing education units through seminars, conferences, and/or other educational means.

For complete details contact:

> Certification of Insurance Rehabilitation Specialists Commission
> 1835 Rohlwing Road, Suite E
> Rolling Meadows, IL 60008
> (847) 394-2106

Professional *Organizations and Suggested Journals*

This appendix includes information about various professional organizations that promote education, support, and standards for the practicing nurse case manager. In addition to the listed national organizations, many states have local organizations that provide the case manager with educational opportunities and large networks of service providers.

American Nurses Association (ANA)
600 Maryland Avenue SW, Suite 100 W
Washington, DC 20024-2571
(800) 284-2378

Official journal: *American Journal of Nursing*
Published by: American Nurses Association
PO Box 50480
Boulder, CO 80322-0480

State Nurses Associations

Alabama State Nurses Association
360 North Hull Street
Montgomery, Alabama 36104-3658
(334) 262-8321

Alaska Nurses Association
237 East Third Avenue
Anchorage, Alaska 99501
(907) 274-0827

ANA/California
P O Box 225,
3010 Wilshire Boulevard
Los Angeles, California 90010
(213) 486-6555

Arkansas Nurses Association
117 South Cedar Street
Little Rock, Arkansas 72205
(501) 664-5853

Colorado Nurses Association
5453 East Evans Place
Denver, Colorado 80222
(303) 757-7483, Ext. 13

District of Columbia
   Nurses Association
5100 Wisconsin Avenue NW,
   Suite 306
Washington, DC 20016
(202) 244-2705

Georgia Nurses Association
1362 West Peachtree Street, NW
Atlanta, Georgia 30339
(404) 876-4624

Hawaii Nurses Association
677 Ala Moana Boulevard,
   Suite 301
Honolulu, Hawaii 96813
(808) 521-8361

Illinois Nurses Association
300 South Wacker Drive,
   Suite 2200
Chicago, Illinois 60606
(312) 360-2300

Arizona Nurses Association
1850 East Southern Avenue, Suite 1
Tempe, Arizona 85282
(602) 831-0404

Connecticut Nurses Association
Meritech Business Park
377 Research Parkway, Suite 2D
Meriden, Connecticut 06450
(203) 238-1207

Delaware Nurses Association
2634 Capitol Trail, Suite A
Newark, Delaware 19711
(302) 368-2333

Florida Nurses Association
P O Box 536985
Orlando, Florida 32853-6985
(407) 896-3261

Guam Nurses Association
P O Box CG
Agana, Guam 96910
011 (671) 477-NURS

Idaho Nurses Association
200 North 4th Street, Suite 20
Boise, Idaho 83702-6001
(208) 345-0500

Indiana State Nurses Association
2915 North High School Road
Indianapolis, Indiana 46224
(317) 299-4575

Iowa Nurses Association
1501 42d Street, Suite 471
West Des Moines, Iowa 50266
(515) 225-0495

Kentucky Nurses Association
P O Box 2616
1400 South First Street,
Louisville, Kentucky 40201
(502) 537-2546/2547

Maine State Nurses Association
P O Box 2240
295 Water Street
Augusta, Maine 04338-2240
(207) 622-1057

Massachusetts Nurses Association
340 Turnpike Street
Canton, Massachusetts 02021
(617) 821-4625

Minnesota Nurses Association
1295 Bandana Boulevard, N,
    Suite 140
Saint Paul, Minnesota 55108-5115
(612) 846-4807 (800) 536-4662

Missouri Nurses Association
P O Box 105228
1904 Bubba Lane
Jefferson City, Missouri 65110
(314) 636-4623

Nebraska Nurses Association
1430 South Street, Suite 202
Lincoln, Nebraska 68502-2446
(402) 475-3859

Kansas State Nurses Association
700 SW Jackson, Suite 601
Topeka, Kansas 66603
(913) 233-8638

Louisiana State Nurses Association
712 Transcontinental Drive
Metairie, Louisiana 70001
(504) 889-1030

Maryland Nurses Association
849 International Drive
Airport Square 21, Suite 255
Linthicum, Maryland 21090
(410) 859-3000

Michigan Nurses Association
2310 Jolly Oak Road
Okemos, Michigan 48864-4599
(517) 349-5640

Mississippi Nurses Association
135 Bounds Street, Suite 100
Jackson, Mississippi 39206
(601) 982-9182

Montana Nurses Association
P O Box 5718
104 Broadway, Suite G-2
Helena, Montana 59601
(406) 442-6710

Nevada Nurses Association
3660 Baker Lane, Suite 104
Reno, Nevada 89509
(702) 825-3555

New Hampshire
  Nurses Association
48 West Street
Concord, New Hampshire 03301
(603) 225-3783

New Mexico Nurses Association
909 Virginia, NE, Suite 101
Albuquerque, New Mexico 87108
(505) 268-7744

North Carolina Nurses Association
Box 12025
103 Enterprise Street,
Raleigh, North Carolina 27605
(919) 821-4250

Ohio Nurses Association
4000 East Main Street
Columbus, Ohio 43213-2950
(614) 237-5414

Oregon Nurses Association
9600 SW Oak, Suite 550
Portland, Oregon 97223
(503) 293-0011

Rhode Island State
  Nurses Association
550 South Water Street, Unit 540B
Providence,
  Rhode Island 02903-4334
(401) 421-9703

South Dakota Nurses Association
1505 South Minnesota Avenue,
  Suite 6
Sioux Falls, South Dakota 57105
(605) 338-1401

New Jersey State
  Nurses Association
320 West State Street
Trenton, New Jersey 08618
(609) 392-4884

New York State Nurses Association
46 Cornell Road
Latham, New York 12110
(518) 782-9400

North Dakota Nurses Association
549 Airport Road
Bismarck, North Dakota 58504-6107
(701) 223-1385

Oklahoma Nurses Association
6414 North Santa Fe, Suite A
Oklahoma City, Oklahoma 73116
(405) 840-3476

Pennsylvania Nurses Association
P O Box 68525
2578 Interstate Drive,
Harrisburg,
  Pennsylvania 17106-8525
(717) 657-1222

South Carolina Nurses Association
1821 Gadsden Street
Columbia, South Carolina 29201
(803) 252-4781

Tennessee Nurses Association
545 Mainstream Drive, Suite 405
Nashville, Tennessee 37228-1201
(615) 254-0350

Texas Nurses Association
7600 Burnel Road, Suite 440
Austin, Texas 78757-1292
(512) 452-0645

Vermont State Nurses Association
PO Box 26, Champlain Mill,
1 Main Street
Winooski, Vermont 05404-2230
(802) 655-7123

Virginia Nurses Association
7113 Three Chopl Road, Suite 204
Richmond, Virginia 23226
(804) 282-1808/2373

West Virginia Nurses Association
2003 Quarrier Street
Charleston,
   West Virginia 25311-4911
(304) 342-1169

Wyoming Nurses Association
Majestic Building, Room 305
1603 Capitol Avenue
Cheyenne, Wyoming 82001
(307) 635-3955

Utah Nurses Association
455 East 400 South, Suite 402
Salt Lake City, Utah 84111
(801) 322-3439

Virgin Islands State
   Nurses Association
PO Box 583
St. Croix,
   U.S. Virgin Islands 00820-4355
(809) 773-2323, Ext. 119/116

Washington State
   Nurses Association
2505 Second Avenue, Suite 500
Seattle, Washington 98121
(206) 443-9762

Wisconsin Nurses Association
8117 Monona Drive
Madison, Wisconsin 53716
(608) 221-0383

Association of Managed Healthcare Organizations (AMHO)
1101 Connecticut Avenue NW, Suite 700
Washington, DC 20036

Official journal: *Health Care Innovations*
Published by: Health Care Communications, Inc. (HCC)
One Bridge Plaza, Suite 350
Fort Lee, NJ 07024
(201) 947-5545

Association of Rehabilitation Nurses (ARN)
4700 W. Lake Avenue
Glenview, IL 60025-1485
(800) 229-7530

Official journal: *Rehabilitation Nursing*
Published by: The Association of Rehabilitation Nurses

Case Management Society of America (CMSA)
8201 Cantrell Road, Suite 230
Little Rock, AR 72227-2448
(501) 225-2229

Official journal: *The Journal of Care Management*
Published by: Mason Medical Communications, Inc.
35 E. Main Street
Westport, CT 06880
(203) 454-2300

Individual Case Management Association (ICMA)
7250 Parkway Drive, Suite 510
Hanover, MD 21076
(800) 664-2620

Official journal: *The Case Manager*
Published by: Mosby-Year Book, Inc.
11830 Westline Industrial Drive
St. Louis, MO 63146-3318
(800) 453-4351

National Association of Professional Geriatric Care Managers (NAPGCM)
1604 North Country Club Road
Tucson, AZ 85716
(520) 881-8008

National Association of Rehabilitation Professionals in the Private Sector (NARPPS)
313 Washington Street, #302
Newton, MA 02158
(617) 692-2035

Other Journals

Business Insurance
Crain Communications, Inc.
740 North Rush Street
Chicago, IL 60611-2590
(800) 678-9595

Case Review, The Journal for
    Case Management Professionals
Allied Health Care Publications
4676 Admiralty Way, Suite 202
Marina del Rey, CA 90292
(310) 306-2206

Inside Case Management
Aspen Publishers, Inc.
7201 McKinney Circle
Frederick, MD 21701
(301) 417-7500

Journal of Rehabilitation
633 South Washington Street
Alexandria, VA 22314

Journal of Subacute Care
Integrated Health Services, Inc.
10065 Red Run Blvd.
Owings Mills, MD 21117
(800) 582-7050

Case Manager Advisor
American Health Consultants
3525 Piedmont Road, NE
Building Six, Suite 400
Atlanta, GA 30305
(404) 262-7436

Continuing Care
Stevens Publishing Corporation
3700 IH-35
Waco, TX 76706
(817) 776-9000

Journal of Nursing Administration
Aspen Publishers, Inc.
7201 McKinney Circle
Frederick, MD 21701
(301) 417-7500

Journal of Rehabilitation
    Research and Development
Superintendent of Documents
U.S. Government Printing
    Office (GPO)
Washington, DC 20402
Stock Number 051-000-00175-3

Risk Management
Risk Management Society
    Publishing Inc.
205 East 42nd Street
New York, NY 10017
(212) 286-9364

A Week in the Life of a Case Manager

This appendix is a diary of a typical week in the life of an external case manager. For the purpose of clarity, only one client will be discussed. The reader should remember that the average external case manager works with about 20 to 30 clients at the same time.

This case is about Carol Peterson, a 40-year-old female who was diagnosed with breast cancer 1 year ago. She has been an inpatient at Mercy Hospital for 3 months due to multiple complications. Although case management has been shown to be most beneficial and effective with early referral, this client was not referred by the insurance company for case management services until 1 year following initial diagnosis.

MONDAY

9:00 A.M.

I receive a phone call from Priya Bhatt, RN, a case manager at Triangle Insurance Company. She is assigning Mrs. Peterson to on-site case management to coordinate a discharge plan from the hospital to a more cost-effective facility. Priya doesn't have any recent information regarding current medical status or the physician's treatment plan or prognosis. She requests that I visit Mrs. Peterson as soon as possible and faxes the referral sheet with the following information:

- Client's name, address, phone number, date of birth
- Policy number and social security number
- Physician's name, address, and phone number
- Name and phone number of Victoria James, the discharge planner at Mercy Hospital
- Diagnosis—breast cancer with metastasis to the lung and spine

9:30 A.M.

I call Victoria James and introduce myself as the on-site case manager, representing Triangle Insurance Company. We arrange for an appointment for the following day at 10:30 A.M. Victoria tells me that she will inform Mrs. Peterson about the visit and will request that Mr. Peterson be in attendance also.

TUESDAY

10:30 A.M.

I meet Victoria James in her office and briefly discuss my role as case manager. She is informed that we will be working together to coordinate a timely, cost-effective discharge plan. Victoria is told that any questions regarding insurance coverage should be directed to my attention.

11:00 A.M.

Victoria and I enter Mrs. Peterson's room and find her awake, alert, oriented, and sitting up in bed. Mr. Peterson is also present, as well as Mrs. Peterson's mother, Mrs. Brown. Victoria introduces me and states she will return in about an hour. I begin by explaining my role and informing Mr. and Mrs. Peterson that use of my services is strictly voluntary. I explain that there is no cost to them for my services and that case management is provided through the insurance carrier as a means of providing high-quality, cost-effective care. I explain that I do not work directly for the carrier but represent it as an independent consultant. After reviewing my role, and answering some basic questions, I request that Mrs. Peterson sign a consent for release of medical information. I explain that the signed release will allow me to review her medical chart and discuss her diagnosis, prognosis, and treatment plan with her physician and will acknowledge that she agrees to the case management services.

Mr. Peterson reviews the consent and states that he and his wife are very anxious to receive assistance and have been very frustrated in their attempts to work with "the system." Mrs. Peterson signs the consent after I am satisfied that she and her husband understand my role.

I spend the next hour assessing Mrs. Peterson's current status and treatment, past medical history, socioeconomic status, and support system as well as her specific needs and desires for discharge. Mrs. Peterson, who is quite knowledgeable and a good historian, reports that she was first diagnosed after a routine mammography, slightly more than 1 year ago. She underwent a left radical mastectomy, radiation, and chemotherapy. Approximately 4 months ago, she began to experience severe back pain. An MRI showed that the cancer had metastasized to her spine. She was admitted to Mercy Hospital for another round of chemotherapy.

Over the past 3 months, Mrs. Peterson has had multiple complications, including sepsis, respiratory insufficiency, nausea and vomiting, and intractable pain. Approximately 6 weeks ago, she was diagnosed with congestive heart failure, had to be placed on a ventilator, and spent 3 weeks in the intensive care unit. During that time she had a central line inserted and was placed on hyperalimentation.

About a week ago, Mrs. Peterson began complaining of headaches and blurred vision. She had an MRI of the head that morning and was waiting to speak with her physician, Dr. Lisa Petrillo, to find out the results. Mrs. Peterson becomes increasingly anxious and begins crying, saying, "All I want is to go home." I encourage her to express her feelings, acknowledging how important is her wish to go home, and tell her that I will find out what her home care coverage is, and, if we can do it, I will coordinate her discharge to home as soon as Dr. Petrillo decides that she is medically stable.

I discuss what support system would be available, if we were able to arrange for home care. Mr. Peterson informs me that he is an accountant and works from home. He would be available to assist with his wife's care. Mrs. Brown, who is a spry 68 year old, said that she would be able to assist in her daughter's care as well. Mrs. Brown informs me that she has been staying at her daughter's house to care for her two young grandchildren, ages 8 and 10.

12:15 P.M.

Victoria is back from her morning rounds and asks if I would like to review Mrs. Peterson's chart. I excuse myself and spend the next 45 minutes at the nurse's station, reviewing the chart and discussing a viable discharge plan with Victoria. Victoria has not had an opportunity to discuss the MRI results with Dr. Petrillo and is unaware of the doctor's continued treatment plan. I tell Victoria that I will be in contact with the insurance carrier and with Dr. Petrillo and that I will call her the following day.

1:00 P.M.

I return to Mrs. Peterson's room, explain that I will be speaking with the insurance company and Dr. Petrillo and that I will contact Mr. Peterson the following day.

2:00 P.M.

I call Dr. Petrillo, who is unavailable. I speak with the office manager and introduce myself as Mrs. Peterson's case manager. I am told that Dr. Petrillo will return my call later that day.

4:00 P.M.

I receive a call from Dr. Petrillo, who states that the MRI showed metastasis to the brain. She inquires about hospice benefits and informs me that Mrs. Peterson's prognosis is grave. Her treatment plan is for palliative treatment only. The goals are to arrange for discharge to home as soon as possible and to make Mrs. Peterson as comfortable and pain free as possible, with the following care in place:

1. At least 16 hours of skilled nursing.
2. IV supplies and equipment for hydration. The order will be for D5NS with potassium, multivitamins, and morphine sulfate added to 1000cc, to run over 24 hours. Mrs. Peterson has been tolerating Ensure by mouth and will not be needing continued hyperalimentation at home.
3. Sterile dressing changes to the central line site twice weekly.
4. Chemistry profile with magnesium level to be drawn twice weekly. The results should be faxed to Dr. Petrillo.

I tell Dr. Petrillo that I will verify the patient's hospice and home care benefits and will contact her the following day to obtain any necessary prescriptions.

4:30 P.M.

I call Priya Bhatt and give her a verbal status with the information obtained from the medical chart, Dr. Petrillo, and Mr. and Mrs. Peterson. Priya tells me that she will familiarize herself with Mrs. Peterson's benefits and will speak with me the following morning.

WEDNESDAY

9:30 A.M.

I receive a call from Priya. She informs me that Mrs. Peterson has hospice coverage, but it is limited to $110 per day, which will not be sufficient to cover all her needs. Priya suggests transferring Mrs.

Peterson to a subacute facility. I inform Priya that I will research the cost of a subacute facility, as well as the total cost involved if we arrange for home care.

9:45 A.M.

I contact three subacute facilities in the area and speak with the person in the admissions department to discuss cost. After describing the patient's needs for skilled and unskilled nursing, the cost quoted ranges from $750 per day to $850 per day.

10:45 A.M.

I contact three home care companies in the area and speak with the respective directors of nursing to discuss Mrs. Peterson's needs, hospice coverage, and prognosis. Universal Nurses, Inc. is networked with an IV company and a pharmacy. Staff there are able to quote me a negotiated cost of $675 per day, which includes 16 hours of skilled nursing care and all IV and medication needs.

12:00 NOON

I contact three DME companies in the area and get negotiated costs for a hospital bed, bedside table, bedside commode, standard wheelchair, chux, and unsterile gloves. The negotiated costs are as follows:

Semielectric hospital bed: $100 per month
Commode: $25.00 per month
Bedside table: $20.00 per month
Wheelchair: $40.00 per month
Case of chux: $39.00
Gloves: $8.00

The total cost of home care, including the rental of equipment, would total approximately $700 per day.

1:30 P.M.

I call Priya and discuss the cost of home care and the cost of subacute. Priya is aware that Mrs. Peterson's wish is to return home and, between Mr. Peterson and Mrs. Brown, it was unlikely that additional home care needs would occur. Priya tells me that she will speak with the person in the benefits department to get approval for "out-of-contract" coverage. (Note: The policy allows for $110 per day home care, under the hospice benefits. I am trying to coordinate a more costly and comprehensive home care discharge plan. I am attempting to convince the insurance carrier that the cost of home care will be equivalent to, and possibly less than, subacute, and will give the patient the opportunity to return home, which is her wish.)

1:45 P.M.

I call Victoria and inform her that I am trying to arrange for home care, provided that the insurance carrier will cover the necessary equipment, supplies, and nursing care. Victoria tells me that she will speak with Mrs. Peterson and let her know that I will contact Mr. Peterson as soon as I have a definite answer from the carrier.

2:00 P.M.

I call Dr. Petrillo to review the potential coverage and projected discharge plan. She approves the plan and requests that I call her as soon as I have a definite answer. In the meantime, for time effectiveness, she faxes me prescriptions for all the IV, medications, and orders for nurses.

4:00 P.M.

I receive a phone call from Priya stating that the person in benefits agreed to provide out-of-contract coverage for 30 days. At the end of the 30 days, the patient's needs and status would be reevaluated for continued coverage. I am also informed that transportation from hospital to home will be covered.

4:15 P.M.

I call Dr. Petrillo and inform her of the available coverage. She asks me if I can arrange all the patient's needs by Friday for discharge Friday afternoon. I assure her that a Friday discharge date would be possible and that I will inform Mrs. Peterson that she will be able to return home before the weekend.

4:30 P.M.

I call Victoria and relate the information concerning the available coverage and a projected discharge date of Friday afternoon. I tell Victoria that I will call Mr. Peterson as soon as we hang up.

4:45 P.M.

I call Mr. Peterson and inform him of the current plan to discharge his wife Friday afternoon. He expresses his appreciation and states that he will not have any problem caring for his wife with the additional assistance from his mother-in-law and close friends. I tell him that he should call me if there are any problems at all, or if he just wants to speak with someone.

4:55 P.M.

I call Universal Nurses, Inc. and inform them that the discharge date is set for Friday. I let them know that I will call them in the morning to discuss the details and fax them the necessary prescriptions. The nursing director assures me that she will coordinate all the IV and medication needs through her network. She is given all the insurance information and the patient's address and phone number.

THURSDAY

9:00 A.M.

I call the DME provider and order the bed, commode, bedside table, wheelchair, chux, and gloves. I give him the insurance information, the patient's name, address, and phone number, and request that he contact Mr. Peterson to arrange for delivery later that day or early Friday morning.

9:30 A.M.

I fax a letter to the DME provider documenting the items to be delivered and the negotiated cost. I fax a copy of the letter to Priya at the insurance company.

10:00 A.M.

I contact Universal Nurses, Inc. and speak with the nursing director. I am told that all shifts through the weekend are covered, starting at 3:00 P.M. on Friday. In addition, all the IV and medication needs have been coordinated and are due to be delivered to Mr. Peterson's home later that day. The IV nurse will be going to the Peterson home for the purpose of teaching and is scheduled to arrive at about 3:30 Friday afternoon. Since the family members will be without nursing coverage for 8 hours daily, it is important that they understand how the IV is set up, how to trouble-shoot in the event of a problem, and how to differentiate between a minor problem and an emergency situation. In addition, it is important for the family members to know how to change the dressing to the central line site, in the event the dressing becomes soiled during their time without nursing assistance.

10:15 A.M.

I fax a letter to the nursing agency documenting the agreed upon nursing care and cost, as well as the IV and medication needs and cost. I include that approval is for 30 days, to be reevaluated at that time. A copy of the letter is faxed to Priya.

10:45 A.M.

I call three patient transportation companies for cost comparison and arrange for stretcher transport with a provider that I have used many times. He quotes me a negotiated cost and faxes me documentation of the arrangements. I give him the insurance information and Mrs. Peterson's hospital room number and request that he pick up the patient at 1:00 P.M. Friday. I then fax a copy of his documentation to Priya.

11:00 A.M.

I call Victoria and inform her that transportation is arranged for a 1:00 P.M. pickup the following day. She tells me that she will inform Mr. and Mrs. Peterson that everything is coordinated for discharge the next day. I ask Victoria to call me Friday morning if there is any change in status or plans.

11:15 A.M.

I call Dr. Petrillo and speak with the office manager. I ask that she inform Dr. Petrillo that everything is coordinated for a 1:00 P.M.

discharge Friday. I request that either she or the doctor contact me with any changes in the plan.

11:30 A.M.

I contact Priya to inform her that everything is in place for a Friday afternoon discharge. She states that she received all the faxes with documented costs and services and has given the appropriate information to the people in the benefits department.

FRIDAY

9:30 A.M.

I call Mr. Peterson, who informs me that all the DME and supplies were delivered Thursday evening. He is anxious to have his wife home and will be going to the hospital to wait with her for the ambulance transport. He is aware that the pickup time is scheduled for 1:00. I tell Mr. Peterson that the first shift of nurses is scheduled to begin at 3:00 that afternoon. I tell him that I will call again later in the day, to make sure everything is going smoothly.

1:30 P.M.

I call Victoria, who informs me that Mrs. Peterson was already picked up and should be arriving home shortly. I thank her for all her assistance and let her know that I will be continuing to provide case management services for Mrs. Peterson at home, to continue coordinating her care as her needs may change.

4:30 P.M.

I call Mr. Peterson, who informs me that the nurse arrived at 3:00 and the IV nurse came in at about 3:30. Everything appears to be in place.

Mrs. Peterson is very happy to be home and is sleeping comfortably. I tell Mr. Peterson that if any problems should arise during the weekend, he should call the nursing agency, which has somebody on call 24 hours per day, 7 days per week. I tell him that I will call him Monday morning to see how the weekend went.

4:45 P.M.

I call Priya and inform her that Mrs. Peterson is at home, resting comfortably, and that everything went smoothly. I inform her that she will receive my initial report the following week.

DISCUSSION

If this were a real client, the case manager would submit a lengthy initial report documenting all the activity that occurred during the discharge planning process (similar to Appendix I reports). A cost-benefit analysis would be included, documenting the authorized care, regular cost, negotiated cost, and cost savings from all the providers involved (see Table A-1).

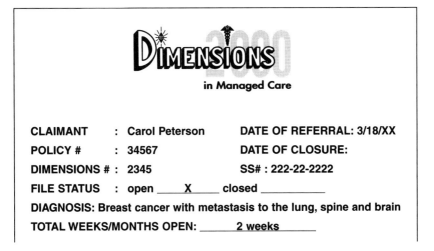

DIMENSIONS 2000
in Managed Care

CLAIMANT : Carol Peterson	**DATE OF REFERRAL: 3/18/XX**	
POLICY # : 34567	**DATE OF CLOSURE:**	
DIMENSIONS # : 2345	**SS# : 222-22-2222**	
FILE STATUS : open ___X___ closed _____		

DIAGNOSIS: Breast cancer with metastasis to the lung, spine and brain

TOTAL WEEKS/MONTHS OPEN: _____2 weeks_____

SUMMARY OF CASE MANAGEMENT INTERVENTION

Coordinated time-effective, cost-effective discharge from acute care to home.
Provided support and encouragement.

Hard Savings

Item/Service	Regular Cost	Negotiated Cost	Savings
Supplies			
Unsterile gloves	$19.20 (2 bxs)	$16.00	$ 3.20
Case of chux	$46.80	$39.00	$ 7.80
Nursing care			
LPN	$37.00/hr × 16 hr/day × 2 wk = $8288.00	$32.00/hr × 16 hr/day × 2 wk = $7168.00	$1120.00
RN high-tech visit (to draw blood)	$125.00/vs × 2/wk = $500.00	$95.00/vs × 2/wk = $380.00	$ 120.00
IV supplies			
D5NS with meds, supplies and IV pole	$110.00/day × 14 days = $1540.00	$86.13/day × 14 days = $1205.82	$ 334.18
DME			
Semielectric hospital bed	$120.00/mo	$100.00/mo	$ 20.00/mo
Commode	$30.00/mo	$25.00/mo	$ 5.00/mo
Wheelchair	$48.00/mo	$40.00/mo	$ 8.00/mo
Bedside table	$50.40/mo	$42.00/mo	$ 8.40/mo
Transportation	$185.00	$158.00	$ 27.00

Subacute	$750.00/day × 14 days = $10,500.00		
Home care		$640.00/day × 14 days = $8960.00	$1540.00
Totals	$10,827.40 home care or $10,500.00 subacute	$10,757.82 home care or $8960.00 subacute	$3193.58 home care over subacute

Potential charges (this report period): $10,827.40 (home care without case management, or $10,500.00 if patient transferred to subacute)

Actual charges (this report period): $10,757.82

Total savings (this report period): $3193.58

Case management fees (to date): $750.00

Net savings: $2443.58

$3.26 saved for every dollar spent

The case manager would maintain contact with the client and her husband, the physician, and the nursing director to assess the client's changing needs and status. After the first 30 days, the case manager would contact the insurance case manager to discuss approval for continued benefits at home. If the client's husband found it was too difficult to care for his wife, or if the cost of home care became more expensive due to the need for additional skilled nursing hours, the insurance carrier may decide not to continue with extracontractual coverage. If that were to happen, the case manager would assist in coordinating a transfer to a more cost-effective subacute facility.

As you can see, the case manager visited with the patient on only one occasion. The majority of the work was done by telephone. It is important to realize that through case management the patient was able to go home to die, which was her wish. Had a case manager not been involved, Mrs. Peterson would have been transferred from the acute care hospital to a less costly subacute facility. She would not have been able to return home and be around her family and children.

The "hands-on" nurses were able to give Mrs. Peterson emotional support and encouragement to verbalize, which she needed for acceptance and closure. The physician was able to prescribe the medications that would alleviate the pain. Mr. Peterson and the children were able to provide an environment of love and support. The nurse case manager, through creative use of her skills and knowledge, enabled Mrs. Peterson to satisfy her one desire—to die at home.

Critical Pathways VI

A *critical pathway*, also referred to as a *clinical pathway* or a *MAP* (multidisciplinary action plan), has become the accepted guide for standardizing treatment and measuring outcomes. Designed as a grid along a timeline, the critical pathway outlines events which are expected to occur at a specific point in the treatment episode. If the outcome is not achieved, it is documented as a variance.

Most facilities develop and design critical pathways specific to the individual needs of the institution. This appendix gives examples of critical pathways that are used in specific acute care hospitals for the following conditions:

Congestive heart failure
Pneumonia
Total hip replacement

Table VI.1 Congestive Heart Failure: CareMap

Location	Day 1 ER 1–4 Hours	Day 1 Floor Telemetry/CCU 6–24 Hours	Day 2 Floor	Day 3 Floor	Day 4 Floor	Day 5 Floor	Day 6 Floor
Problem							
1. Alteration in gas exchange/profusion and fluid balance due to decreased cardiac output excess fluid volume.	Reduce pain from admission or pain free. Uses pain scale. O_2 sat. improved over admission baseline on O_2 therapy.	Respirations equal to or less than on admission.	O_2 sat = 90. Resp 20–22. Vital signs stable. Crackles at lung bases. Mild shortness of breath with activity.	Does not require O_2. Vital signs stable. Crackles at bases. Resp. 20–22. Mild shortness of breath with activity.	Does not require O_2. (O_2 sat. on room air 90%.) Vital signs stable. Crackles at bases. Resp. 20–22. Completes activities with no increase in respirations. No edema.	Can lie in bed at baseline position. Chest X-ray clear or at baseline.	No dyspnea.
2. Potential for shock.	No signs/symptoms of shock.	No signs/symptoms of shock.	No signs/symptoms of shock.	No signs/symptoms of shock. Normal lab values.	No signs/symptoms of shock.	No signs/symptoms of shock.	No signs/symptoms of shock.

3. Potential for consequences of immobility and decreased activity: skin breakdown, DVT.	No redness at pressure points. No falls.	No redness at pressure points. No falls.	Tolerates chair, washing, eating, and toileting.	Has bowel movement. Up in room and bathroom with assist.	Up ad lib for short periods.	Activity increased to level used at home without shortness of breath.	Activity increased to level used at home without shortness of breath.
4. Alteration in nutritional intake due to nausea and vomiting.		No c/o nausea. No vomiting. Taking liquids as offered.	Eating solids. Takes in 50% each meal.	Taking 50% each meal.	Taking 50% each meal. Weight 2 lbs. from patient's normal baseline.	Taking 75% each meal.	Taking 75% each meal.
5. Potential for arrhythmias due to decreased cardiac output, decreased irritable foci, valve problems, gas exch. →	No evidence of life-threatening dysrhythmias.	Normal sinus rhythm with benign ectopy.	K+ (WNL). Benign or no arrhythmias.	Digoxin level WNL. Benign or no arrhythmias.	Digoxin level WNL. Benign or no arrhythmias.	Digoxin level WNL. Benign or no arrhythmias.	Digoxin level WNL. Benign or no arrhythmias.

Continued on next page

Table VI.1 Congestive Heart Failure: CareMap *Continued*

	Day 1	Day 1	Day 2	Day 3	Day 4	Day 5	Day 6
6. Patient/family response to future treatment & hospitalization.		Patient/family expressing concerns. Following directions of staff.	Patient/family expressing concerns. Following directions of staff.	Patient/family expressing concerns. Following directions of staff.	States reasons for and cooperates with rest periods. Patient begins to assess own knowledge and ability to care for CHF at home.	Patient decides whether he/she wants discussion with physician about advanced directives.	States plan for 1–2 days post discharge as to meds., diet, activity, follow-up appointments. Expresses reaction to having CHF.
Staff Tasks							
Assessment/Consults	Vital signs q15min. Nursing assessments focus on lung sounds, edema, color, skin integrity, jugular vein distention. Cardiac monitor, arterial line if needed Swan Ganz, intake & output.	Vital signs q15min–1 h. Repeat nursing assessments. Cardiac monitor, arterial line, Swan Ganz. Daily weight. Intake & output.	Vital signs q4h. Repeat nursing assessments. D/C cardiac monitor 24h. D/C arterial + Swan Ganz. Daily weight. Intake & output.	Vital signs q6h Repeat nursing assessments. Daily weight. Intake & output.	Vital signs q6h. Repeat nursing assessments. Daily weight. Intake & output. Nutrition consult.	Vital signs q6h. Repeat nursing assessments. Daily weight. Intake & output.	Vital signs q6h. Repeat nursing assessments. Daily weight. Intake & output.

Specimens/Tests	Consider TSH studies. Chest X-ray, EKG, CPK—8 hr × 3, ABG if pulse Ox: (range) Lytes. Na. K. Cl., CO_2 Glucose, BUN, Creatinine, Digoxin: (range)	B/G	Evaluate for ECHO. Lytes, BUN, Creatinine.		Chest X-ray. Lytes, BUN, Creatinine.
Treatments	O_2 or intubate. IV or Hep lock.	O_2 IV or Hep lock	IV or Hep lock	DC pulse Ox if stable. D/C IV/Hep lock.	

Continued on next page

Table VI.1 Congestive Heart Failure: CareMap *Continued*

Staff Tasks *cont.*	Day 1	Day 1	Day 2	Day 3	Day 4	Day 5	Day 6
Medications	Evaluate for Digoxin, Nitrodrip or paste, Diuretics IV. Evaluate for antiemetics. Evaluate for antiarrhythmias.	Evaluate for Digoxin, Nitrodrip or paste, Diuretics IV. Evaluate for preload/after-load reducers, K supplements, Stool softeners.	D/C Nitrodrip or paste, Diuretics, IV or PO. K supplements. Stool softeners. Evaluate for nicotine patch.	Change to PO Digoxin. PO diuretics. K supplements. Stool softeners. Nicotine patch if consent.	PO diuretics. K supplement. Stool softeners. Nicotine patch if consent.	PO diuretics. K supplement. Stool softeners. Nicotine patch if consent.	PO diuretics. K supplement. Stool softeners. Nicotine patch if consent.
Nutrition	None	Clear liquids	Cardiac, low-salt diet	Cardiac, low-salt diet	Cardiac, low-salt diet	Cardiac, low-salt diet	
Safety/ Activity	Commode. Bedrest with head elevated. Reposition patient q2h. Bedrails up. Call light available.	Commode. Bedrest with head elevated. Dangle. Reposition patient q2h. Enforce rest periods. Bedrails up. Call light available.	Commode. Enforce rest periods. Chair with assist. ½ hr. with feet elevated. Bedrails up. Call light available.	Bathroom privileges. Chair × 3. Bedrails up. Call light available.	Ambulate in hall × 2. Up ad lib between rest periods. Bedrails up. Call light available.	Encourage ADLs that approximate activities at home. Bedrails up. Call light available.	Encourage ADLs that approximate activities at home. Bedrails up. Call light available.

Teaching	Explain procedures. Teach chest pain scale and importance of reporting.	Explain course, need for energy conservation. Orient to unit and routine.	Clarify CHF Dx and future teaching needs. Orient to unit and routine. Schedule rest periods. Begin medication teaching.	Importance of weighing self every day. Provide smoking cessation information. Review energy conservation schedule.	Cardiac rehab level as indicated by consult. Provide smoking cessation support. Dietary teaching.	Review CHF education material with patient.	Reinforce CHF teaching.
Transfer/ Discharge Coordination	Assess home situation: notify significant other. If no arrhythmias or chest pain, transfer to floor, otherwise transfer to ICU.	Screen for discharge needs. Transfer to floor.	Consider Home Health Care referral.		Evaluate needs for diet and anti-smoking classes. Physician offers discussion opportunities for advanced directives.	Appointment and arrangements for follow-up care with Home Health Care nurses. Contact VNA.	Reinforce follow-up appointments.

Source: By permission from The Center for Case Management, South Natick, MA

Table VI.2 Congestive Heart Failure: Critical Pathway at St. Michael Hospital, Milwaukee, WI

	Day 1	Day 2	Day 3	Day 4	Day 5	Day 6–7
Documentation	Working Doc. and Treatment Plan.					Final Doc. when possible.
Floor	MCU/2N with telemetry.	2N with telemetry.			DC telemetry.	
Consults	Assess Need: Cardiologist.	Assess Need: Dietitian, O.T. for energy conservation.				
Tests	CXR. EKG. Lytes. Chem. Profile Assess Need: Cardiac enzymes.	CXR. EKG. Lytes. Assess Need: Dig. level. Echo.	CXR. Lytes.	BUN. Creat.		
Activity	Commode PRN. Bedrest.			Up in chair.	Up in hall.	
Treatments	Daily weights. I&O. Foley, VS–q 4°. IV or Hep lock.	Daily weights. I&O. Foley. VS BID/PRN. Hep lock.	Daily weights. I&O. DC Foley. Hep lock.	Daily weights. I&O. Hep lock.	Daily weights. I&O. Hep lock.	Daily weights. I&O. Hep lock.

					Discharge. Complete multi-disciplinary. Discharge teaching record.
Medications	O$_2$, IV Diuretic, Analgesia, Assess Need: Nitrates, Dobutamine.	O$_2$, IV Diuretic, Assess Need: K+ supplement.	DC O$_2$ or PRN. Oral diuretics.		
Diet	NAS (Assess need for cholesterol and weight loss).				
Discharge/ Planning	Database & assessment of home care situation.		Assess DC needs & date. Contact SS/HH.		DC orders DC meds Follow-up appointment.
Key Nursing Activities/ Teaching	Pt. oriented to room, routine & primary nursing. Assess & Monitor: 1. Head to toe assessment—shift and PRN.	Continue to assess 1-10 BID. Teach A&P of heart: S&S of CHF; importance of daily wgt. & edema record.	Initiate medication instruction. Review diet, activity progression & energy conservation techniques/ work simplification.	Review S&S of CHF, how & when to contact MD with problems.	Review home maintenance program for CHF—meds., diet, activity, follow-up help.

Continued on next page

Table VI.2 Congestive Heart Failure: Critical Pathway at St. Michael Hospital, Milwaukee, WI *Continued*

	Day 1	Day 2	Day 3	Day 4	Day 5	Day 6–7
Key Nursing Activities/ Teaching (*continued*)	2. Skin risk & skin integrity assessment. 3. Activity restriction. 4. Heart sounds. 5. JUD. 6. RR & lung sounds. 7. Diet. 8. EKG/ monitors. 9. K+ levels. 10. Dependent edema. 11. Sleep/rest pat. Teaching. To Pt./Sig. Other CHF teaching packet & book-let, "A Stronger Pump" given. Definition of CHF. Promotion of outlet environ-ment & rest.	Introduction to stress mgmt., relaxation techniques (consider O.T. consult). Provide smoking cessation support if needed.	Reinforce stress mgmt/relax-ation teaching. Orient to CCTV & appropriate programs.			

Key Patient Activities/Outcomes	Pt. demonstrates use of call light. Pt. &/or sig. other verbalizes what CHF means.	Pt. &/or sig. other verbalizes A/P of heart failure. Pt. &/or sig. other begins recording daily weight & edema.	Pt. &/or sig. other verbalizes use of meds., dietary/activity progression balanced with rest re: CHF. Pt. watches CCTV appropriate programs (i.e., stress reduction, relaxation tech. & smoking cessation).	Pt. &/or sig. other verbalizes early warning S&S of CHF & a home plan for contacting emergency help.	Pt. &/or sig. other describes home med. schedule with indications/S.E. (med sheet PRN). Pt. &/or sig. other verbalizes home maintenance programs of CHF: Activity, Diet, Daily Weight, Follow-up appt., Emergency Plans, Access to support programs.

Potential Nursing Diagnoses

*1. Activity intolerance
2. Alteration in cardiac output
3. Knowledge deficit re: CHF, meds

*Indicates standard nursing care guide

WIPRO Criteria—All Met & Documented Before Discharge

72° a DC   24–48° a DC
No evidence of   *Lab values within normal range 24° PTD
EKG PTD   (e.g., K+. BUN, Creat.)
   *Improved clinical status (e.g., stable wt. edema, chest clear of rales & wheezing).

By permission of Mary Therese Sinnen and Marita Mackinnon Schifalacqua.

Table VI.3 Pneumonia

	ER/Day 1	Day 2	Day 3	Day 4	Day 5	Day 6	Day 7
Assessments & Evaluations	Nursing Assessment. VS, Temp & Br. Sq4h. 7–3 ___ 3–11 ___ 11–7 ___ Resp. Assessment. WET Team screen. Case Mgr. Assessment. Dr. to assess code status. (ER): H&P Admit Note Doc. Fall of O.P. Tx. Note of Asp. Event.	Nursing Assessment. VS, Temp & Br. Sq4h. 7–3 ___ 3–11 ___ 11–7 ___ Case Mgr. Assessment. Nutritional screen. Activity Tol. Assessment. Review labs from prev. day.	Nursing Assessment. VS, Temp & Br. Sq4h. 7–3 ___ 3–11 ___ 11–7 ___ Case Mgr. Assessment. Review labs from prev. day.	Nursing Assessment. VS, Temp & Br. Sq4h. 7–3 ___ 3–11 ___ 11–7 ___ If Afebrile–DC VS & Temp q4h. If Br. S improved– DC Br. Sq4h. Case Mgr. Assessment. Review labs from prev. day.	Nursing Assessment. 7–3 ___ 3–11 ___ 11–7 ___ Case Mgr. Assessment. Review labs from prev. day.	Nursing Assessment. 7–3 ___ 3–11 ___ 11–7 ___ Case Mgr. Assessment. Review labs from prev. day.	Nursing Assessment. 7–3 ___ 3–11 ___ 11–7 ___ Case Mgr. Assessment. Review labs from prev. day.

Test	Test results from outside sources acceptable. (ER): CXR— r/o lobar, consol. Sput Cult & GM St. Blood Sugar CBC BUN & Cr RA Pulse Oximetry ABG if SP O_2 < 90% (ERx1) Blood Cult Albumin Level if indicated UA.	Preliminary test results to chart. If CXR has upper lobe infiltrate, consider PPD. If prior PPD pos., then obtain sputum for acid fast GS & C.	Confirm all test results to chart.	Repeat CXR. CBC. Final culture results to chart.	Results on chart. CXR CBC		

Continued on next page

359

Table VI.3 Pneumonia *Continued*

	ER/Day 1	Day 2	Day 3	Day 4	Day 5	Day 6	Day 7
Consults	Order if indicated Pulmonary Inf. Disease WET Team	Evaluate need for: Clin Soc. Worker Geriatric Nurse Spec.					
Treatments	C & DB q2h WA RT Tx. if indicated.	C & DB q2h WA RT Tx. if indicated.	C & DB q2h WA RT Tx. if indicated.	If Br. S Improved– DCq2h C & DB			
Medications	O_2 per protocol. (ER): IV (HL asap) IV Antibiotics after cultures. Cough Rx Order maintenance meds. Consider Heparin DVT Prophylaxis	O_2 if indicated. IV (HL asap) IV Antibiotics Cough Rx Maint. meds.	O_2 if indicated. IV (HL asap) IV Antibiotics Cough Rx Maint. meds. Eval for home IV Tx	IV (HL asap) IV Antibiotics Cough Rx Maint. meds.	Consider PO Antibiotic Cough Rx Maint. meds.	Consider PO Antibiotic Cough Rx Maint. meds.	Consider PO Antibiotic Cough Rx Maint. meds.

	Activity as ordered	Encourage activity to tolerance	Encourage activity to tolerance	Encourage activity to tolerance	Encourage activity to tolerance	Encourage activity to tolerance
Activity	Diet as ordered	Diet as ordered	Diet as ordered	Diet as ordered	Diet as ordered	Diet as ordered
Diet	Diet as ordered	Diet as ordered	Diet as ordered	Diet as ordered	Diet as ordered	Diet as ordered
Elimination	I&O Monitor stools	I&O Monitor stools	I&O Monitor stools	DC I&O DC Monitor stools		
Education	Nursing Instruction: C & DB fluids (as indicated) Handwashing Tissue disposal Fall tips Handout	Reinforce instructions If smoker: stop info. (Lifetrends II) Case Mgr. Instruction: Pneumonia Self-Care	Reinforce instructions	Reinforce instructions	Reinforce instructions Diet Instruction as needed Med. Instruction as needed	Reinforce instructions

Source: By permission: *Inside Case Management.*

361

Table VI.4 Total Hip Replacement

Nursing Diagnosis	Goals	Goals Met at Discharge		
		Yes	No	Nurses' Signature
1. Potential anxiety related to hospitalization and/or surgical procedure.	1. Patient and/or family will verbalize or exhibit decreased anxiety.	1. ___ ___ _____ Date achieved: ___		
2. Potential alteration in tissue and peripheral perfusion.	2. Circulation, sensation, and movement of affected extremity within normal limits.	2. ___ ___ _____ Date achieved: ___		
3. Potential alteration in comfort: pain related to surgery.	3. Pain controlled at time of discharge.	3. ___ ___ _____ Date achieved: ___		
4. Potential alteration in respiratory function related to anesthesia and decreased mobility.	4. Normal respiration pattern for patient.	4. ___ ___ _____ Date achieved: ___		
5. Potential for fluid volume deficit related to blood loss.	5. Adequate hydration, vital signs within normal limits, and balanced intake and output.	5. ___ ___ _____ Date achieved: ___		
6. Potential for infection related to surgical intervention.	6. The patient will be free from infectious process during hospitalization.	6. ___ ___ _____ Date achieved: ___		
7. Potential alteration in skin integrity related to decreased mobility.	7. Patient will be free of areas of skin breakdown and the surgical wound will be healing.	7. ___ ___ _____ Date achieved: ___		
8. Potential impaired physical mobility related to surgical intervention and/or disease process.	8. Patient ambulates safely using assistive devices, verbalizes and/or demonstrates safety in mobility and transfers to avoid injury.	8. ___ ___ _____ Date achieved: ___		

9. Potential altered elimination: constipation related to anesthesia, pain medication, and immobility.

10. Potential altered patterns in urinary elimination related to anesthesia, pain medication, and decreased mobility.

11. Potential alterations in self-care related to decreased mobility and/or disease process.

12. Potential knowledge deficit related to discharge from hospital.

9. Patient returns to normal bowel elimination patterns.

10. Patient returns to normal voiding pattern.

11. Patient will be independent in ADLs with appropriate assistive devices as needed.

12. Patient and/or family verbalizes discharge instructions, and/or able to give return demonstration of treatments and self-care.

9. _____ Date achieved: _____

10. _____ Date achieved: _____

11. _____ Date achieved: _____

12. _____ Date achieved: _____

Additional Problems

13. _____

14. _____

13. _____

14. _____

13. _____ Date achieved: _____

14. _____ Date achieved: _____

Signature	Initials	Signature	Initial	Signature	Initial	Signature	Initial

TUCSON MEDICAL CENTER
DIVISION OF NURSING
TOTAL HIP REPLACEMENT CarePlan MAP©
ORTHOPEDIC TRANSITIONAL CARE UNIT

Table VI. 4 Total Hip Replacement *Continued*

Hospital Day	Consults	Tests	Activity/ Rest	Medical Interventions	Medications	Nutrition	Nurses' Signatures
ADMISSION TO O.T.C.U: Day 1 Date: ____ Post-op day: ____	—Physical Therapy consult[1,12]	—Daily proteins as ordered[2]	—Progressive ambulation with assistance[2,4,7,8,9,11] —Non-weight bearing or as ordered[2,4,7,8,9,11] —Out-of-bed in chair for meals[2,4,7,8,9,11] —Knee strengthening exercises[2,8] —Quad sets QID[2,8] —Ankle pumps, gluteal sets PRN[2,8] —Upper extremity exercises (pull-ups and isometrics)[2,8] —Maintain hip precautions[2,3,8,12] —Assisted abduction 10 to 20 minutes with roller skate QID[2,8] —Pool therapy[2,8] —P.T. routine total hip program[2,7,8,11]	—Incentive spirometer PRN[4] —Ted stockings Remove for skin care every 8 hours[2,7] —SCDs at night and PRN as ordered[2,7]	—Pain meds: p.o.[3] *Give prior to therapy[3,8] —Sleep meds: PRN[3] —Laxative of choice, enema, or suppository PRN[9] —Continue current home medications[12]	—Regular or special diet[5,9]	(7–3) ____ (3–11) ____ (11–7) ____

Hospital Day	Assessment	Discharge Planning	Teaching	Psychosocial	Self-care	Nurses' Signatures
ADMISSION TO O.T.C.U: Day 1 Date: ___ Post-op Day: ___	—Initiate TCU Care Plan MAP©[12] —Admission assessment care plan[12] —Vital signs BID-TID[4,5] —Assess circulation, sensation, and movement every 8 hours and PRN[2]	—Social Service to initiate a physosocial assessment within 24–48 hours of admission[1,12]	—Reinforce Physical Therapy and Occupational Therapy teaching[12]	—Social Service to assess for discharge planning needs within 24 to 48 hours of admission[1,12]	—Assisted care[11] —Hip precautions[2,3,8,12] —Assisted ADLs[11] —Assisted ambulation in hall or to bathroom[2,4,7,8,9,11] —Implement Occupational Therapy's ADLs program[1,12]	___ (7–3) ___ (3–11) ___ (11–7)

*all items not provided as planned.
Enter explanation in the individualization/variance section on the last page.
DRG Number: 209   NRA-456
Expected LOS: ___ days
Developed by J. Nelson, RN, & D. Myers, RN
Revised by J. Nelson, RN 5/93

Page 3 of 6

TUCSON MEDICAL CENTER
DIVISION OF NURSING
TOTAL HIP REPLACEMENT CarePlan MAP©
ORTHOPEDIC TRANSITIONAL CARE UNIT

Independent Actions Based Upon the Human Response to Actual or Potential Problems, cont'd.

Hospital Day	Consults	Tests	Activity/ Rest	Medical Interventions	Medi- cations	Nutrition	Nurses' Signatures
OTCU Day 2 Date: ____	Assessments: • Recreational[1,11] • Psycho-social[1,12] • Pharmacy[3,9,12] • Nutritional (if on special diet)[1,5,9,12] • Occupational Therapy evaluation[1,12]		—Ambulate to dining room[2,4,7,8,9,11] —Ambulate to bathroom (no bedpan or urinal)[2,4,7,8,9,11]	—Continue as Day 1	—Continue as of Admission Day	—Continue as of Admission Day	(7–3) (3–11) (11–7)
OTCU Day 3 Date: ____	⇑	⇑	⇑	⇑	⇑	⇑	(7–3) (3–11) (11–7)
OTCU Day 4 Date: ____	⇑	⇑	⇑	⇑	⇑	⇑	(7–3) (3–11) (11–7)
OTCU Day 5 Date: ____	⇑	⇑	⇑	—Medication for after discharge given with instructions (prescriptions or medications)[11,12]	⇑	⇑	(7–3) (3–11) (11–7)

Hospital Day	Assessment	Discharge Planning	Teaching	Psychosocial	Self-care	Nurses' Signatures
OTCU Day 2 Date: _____	—Continue as of admission	**EVERY THURSDAY:** Patient Care Conference[1,12] —Assess for needed equipment[11]	—Reinforce Physical Therapy and Occupational Therapy teaching[12]	—Develop Care plan goals (psychosocial)[1,12] —Implement Care plan goals (psychosocial)[1,12]	Continue as of admission[2,4,7,8,9,11]	(7–3) _____ (3–11) _____ (11–7) _____
OTCU Day 3 Date: _____	⟹	⟹	⟹	⟹	⟹	(7–3) _____ (3–11) _____ (11–7) _____
OTCU Day 4 Date: _____	⟹	—Equipment for discharge received[11]	⟹	⟹	⟹	(7–3) _____ (3–11) _____ (11–7) _____
OTCU Day 5 Date: _____	⟹	—Outpatient PT scheduled	—Verbal and written discharge instructions given[11,12]	⟹	⟹	(7–3) _____ (3–11) _____ (11–7) _____

*all items not provided as planned.
Enter explanation in the individualization/variance section on the last page.
DRG Number: 209   NRA-456   Expected LOS: _____ days
Developed by J. Nelson, RN, & D. Myers, RN. Revised by J. Nelson, RN 5/93
Page 5 of 6

TUCSON MEDICAL CENTER
DIVISION OF NURSING
TOTAL HIP REPLACEMENT CarePlan MAP©
ORTHOPEDIC TRANSITIONAL CARE UNIT

367

Hospital Day	Consults	Tests	Activity/ Rest	Medical Interventions	Medications	Nutrition	Nurses' Signatures

TUCSON MEDICAL CENTER
DIVISION OF NURSING
TOTAL HIP REPLACEMENT CarePlan MAP©
ORTHOPEDIC TRANSITIONAL CARE UNIT

*all items not provided as planned.
Enter explanation in the individualization/
variance section on the last page.
DRG Number: 209   NRA-456
Expected LOS: ___ days
Developed by J. Nelson, RN, & D. Myers, RN
Revised by J. Nelson, RN 5/93

Independent Actions Based Upon the Human Response to Actual or Potential Problems, cont.				
Date	Individualization/Variation	Cause	Action Taken	Signature

TUCSON MEDICAL CENTER
DIVISION OF NURSING
TOTAL HIP REPLACEMENT CarePlan MAP©
ORTHOPEDIC TRANSITIONAL CARE UNIT

Tools for Assessment of Clients with Central Nervous System Injury

This appendix includes the following assessment tools:

Rancho levels of cognitive functioning
Glasgow coma scale
Sensory levels
Motor levels

VII-1. Rancho Levels of Cognitive Functioning*

I. NO RESPONSE
Patient appears to be in a deep sleep and is completely unresponsive to any stimuli presented to him.

II. GENERALIZED RESPONSE
Patient reacts inconsistently and nonpurposefully to stimuli in a nonspecific manner. Responses are limited in nature and are often the same regardless of stimulus presented. Responses may be physiological changes, gross body movements and vocalization. Responses are likely to be delayed. The earliest response is to deep pain.

---

*Adapted from "Levels of Cognitive Functioning," *Rehabilitation of the Head Injured Adult: Comprehensive Management.* Downey, California, Professional Staff Association of Rancho Los Amigos Hospital, 1979. pp. 8–11.

III. LOCALIZED RESPONSE

Patient reacts specifically but inconsistently to stimuli. Responses are directly related to the type of stimulus presented as in turning head toward a sound or focusing on an object presented. The patient may withdraw an extremity and vocalize when presented with a painful stimulus. He may follow simple commands in an inconsistent, delayed manner, such as closing his eyes, squeezing or extending an extremity. Once external stimuli are removed, he may lie quietly. He may also show a vague awareness of self and body by responding to discomfort by pulling at nasogastric tube or catheter or resisting restraints. He may show a bias toward responding to some persons, especially family and friends, but not to others.

IV. CONFUSED-AGITATED

Patient is in a heightened state of activity with severely decreased ability to process information. He is detached from the present and responds primarily to his own internal confusion. Behavior is frequently bizarre and nonpurposeful relative to his immediate environment. He may cry out or scream out of proportion to stimuli after removal, may show aggressive behavior, attempt to remove restraints or tube or crawl out of bed in a purposeful manner. He does not discriminate among persons or objects and is unable to cooperate directly with treatment efforts. Verbalization is frequently incoherent or inappropriate to the environment. Confabulation may be present; he may be hostile. Gross attention to environment is very brief and selective attention often nonexistent. Being unaware of present events, patient lacks short term recall and may be reacting to past events. He is unable to perform self-care activities without maximum assistance. If not disabled physically, he may perform automatic motor activities such as sitting, reaching and ambulating, as part of his agitated state but not as a purposeful act or on request necessarily.

V.   CONFUSED-INAPPROPRIATE

Patient appears alert and is able to respond to simple commands fairly consistently. However, with increased complexity of commands or lack of any external structure, responses are nonpurposeful, random, or at best, fragmented toward any desired goal. He may show agitated behavior, but not on an internal basis, as in Level IV, but rather as a result of external stimuli and usually out of proportion to the stimulus. He has gross attention to the environment, is highly distractible and lacks ability to focus attention to a specific task without frequent redirection. With structure, he may be able to converse on a social automatic level for short periods of time. Verbalization is often inappropriate; confabulation may be triggered by present events. Memory is severely impaired, with confusion of past and present in reaction to ongoing activity. Patient lacks initiation of functional tasks and often shows inappropriate use of objects without external direction. He may be able to perform previously learned tasks when structured for him, but is unable to learn new information. He responds best to self, body, comfort and often, family members. The patient can usually perform self-care activities with assistance and may accomplish feeding with supervision. Management on the unit is often a problem if the patient is physically mobile, as he may wander off either randomly or with vague intention of "going home."

VI. CONFUSED-APPROPRIATE

Patient shows goal-directed behavior, but is dependent on external input for direction. Response to discomfort is appropriate and he is able to tolerate unpleasant stimuli, e.g., an NG tube when need is explained. He follows simple directions consistently and shows carry-over for tasks he has relearned; e.g., self-care. He is at least supervised with old learning; unable to maximally assist for new learning with little or no carryover. Responses may be incorrect due to memory problems but are appropriate to the situation. They may be delayed to immediate and he shows information with little or no anticipation or prediction of events. Past memories show more depth and detail than recent memory. The patient may show beginning awareness of his situation by realizing he doesn't know an answer. He no longer wanders and is inconsistently disoriented to time and place. Selective attention to tasks may be impaired, especially with difficult tasks and in unstructured settings, but is now functional for common daily activities. He may show vague recognition of some staff and has increased awareness of self, family, and basic needs.

VII.   AUTOMATIC-APPROPRIATE
Patient appears appropriate and oriented with hospital and home settings, goes through daily routine automatically but robot-like, with minimal to absent confusion and has shallow recall of what he has been doing. He shows increased awareness of self, body, family, food, people and interaction in the environment. He has superficial awareness of but lacks insight into his condition, decreased judgement and problem solving and lacks realistic planning for his future. He shows carryover for new learning at a decreased rate. He requires at least minimal supervision for learning and safety purposes. He is independent in self-care activities and supervised in home and community skills for safety. With structure, he is able to initiate tasks or social and recreational activities in which he now has interest. His judgement remains impaired. Prevocational evaluation and counseling may be indicated.

VIII.   PURPOSEFUL-APPROPRIATE
Patient is alert and oriented, is able to recall and integrate past and recent events and is aware of and responsive to his culture. He shows carryover for new learning if acceptable to him and his life role and needs no supervision once activities are learned. Within his physical capabilities, he is independent in home and community skills. Vocational rehabilitation, to determine ability to return as

a contributor to society, perhaps in a new capacity, is indicated. He may continue to show decreases relative to premorbid abilities in quality and rate of processing, abstract reasoning, tolerance for stress and judgement in emergencies or unusual circumstances. His social, emotional and intellectual capacities may continue to be at a decreased level for him, but functional within society.

VII-2. Glasgow Coma Scale

Examiner's Test		Patient's Response	Assigned Score
Eye Opening:	Spontaneous	Opens eyes on own	4
	Speech	Opens eyes when asked to in a loud voice	3
	Pain	Opens eyes when pinched	2
	Pain	Does not open eyes	1
Best Motor Response	Commands	Follows simple commands	6
	Pain	Pulls examiner's hand away when pinched	5
	Pain	Pulls part of body away when examiner pinches patient	4
	Pain	Flexes body inappropriately to pain (decorticate posturing)	3
	Pain	Body becomes rigid in an extended position when examiner pinches victim (decerebrate posturing)	2
	Pain	Has no motor response to pinch	1
Verbal Response (Talking):	Speech	Carries on a conversation correctly and tells examiner where he is, who he is, and the month and year	5
	Speech	Seems confused or disoriented	4
	Speech	Talks so examiner can understand victim but makes no sense	3
	Speech	Makes sounds that examiner can't understand	2
	Speech	Makes no noise	1

VII-3.   Sensory Levels

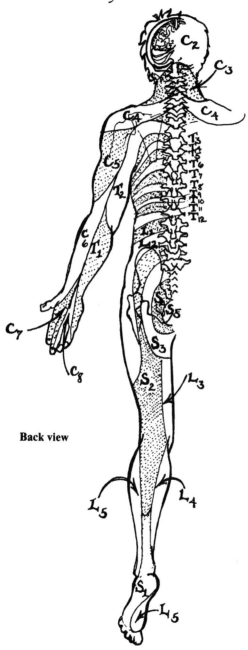

Back view

VII-4.   *Motor Levels*

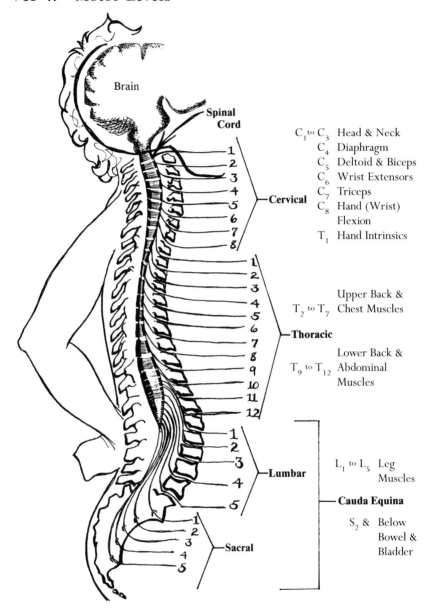

Brain

Spinal Cord

C_1 to C_3 Head & Neck
C_4 Diaphragm
C_5 Deltoid & Biceps
C_6 Wrist Extensors
C_7 Triceps
C_8 Hand (Wrist) Flexion
T_1 Hand Intrinsics

— **Cervical**

T_2 to T_7 Upper Back & Chest Muscles

— **Thoracic**

T_9 to T_{12} Lower Back & Abdominal Muscles

L_1 to L_5 Leg Muscles

— **Lumbar**

— **Cauda Equina**

S_2 &   Below Bowel & Bladder

— **Sacral**

Index

ISBN 0-07-105481-2

90000>

9 780071 054812